Drugs: A Very Short Introduction

'...achieves within a short space an account of the history, the main features of the most commonly used drugs and a peer into the future written in a lively and easily comprehended style.'

Sir Arnold Burgen, Downing College, Cambridge

VERY SHORT INTRODUCTIONS are for anyone wanting a stimulating and accessible way into a new subject. They are written by experts, and have been translated into more than 40 different languages.

The series began in 1995, and now covers a wide variety of topics in every discipline. The VSI library now contains nearly 450 volumes—a Very Short Introduction to everything from Psychology and Philosophy of Science to American History and Relativity—and continues to grow in every subject area.

Very Short Introductions available now:

ACCOUNTING Christopher Nobes
ADOLESCENCE Peter K. Smith
ADVERTISING Winston Fletcher
AFRICAN AMERICAN RELIGION
    Eddie S. Glaude Jr
AFRICAN HISTORY John Parker and
    Richard Rathbone
AFRICAN RELIGIONS Jacob K. Olupona
AGNOSTICISM Robin Le Poidevin
AGRICULTURE Paul Brassley and
    Richard Soffe
ALEXANDER THE GREAT
    Hugh Bowden
ALGEBRA Peter M. Higgins
AMERICAN HISTORY Paul S. Boyer
AMERICAN IMMIGRATION
    David A. Gerber
AMERICAN LEGAL HISTORY
    G. Edward White
AMERICAN POLITICAL HISTORY
    Donald Critchlow
AMERICAN POLITICAL PARTIES
    AND ELECTIONS L. Sandy Maisel
AMERICAN POLITICS
    Richard M. Valelly
THE AMERICAN PRESIDENCY
    Charles O. Jones
THE AMERICAN REVOLUTION
    Robert J. Allison
AMERICAN SLAVERY
    Heather Andrea Williams
THE AMERICAN WEST Stephen Aron
AMERICAN WOMEN'S HISTORY
    Susan Ware

ANAESTHESIA Aidan O'Donnell
ANARCHISM Colin Ward
ANCIENT ASSYRIA Karen Radner
ANCIENT EGYPT Ian Shaw
ANCIENT EGYPTIAN ART AND
    ARCHITECTURE Christina Riggs
ANCIENT GREECE Paul Cartledge
THE ANCIENT NEAR EAST
    Amanda H. Podany
ANCIENT PHILOSOPHY Julia Annas
ANCIENT WARFARE Harry Sidebottom
ANGELS David Albert Jones
ANGLICANISM Mark Chapman
THE ANGLO—SAXON AGE John Blair
THE ANIMAL KINGDOM
    Peter Holland
ANIMAL RIGHTS David DeGrazia
THE ANTARCTIC Klaus Dodds
ANTISEMITISM Steven Beller
ANXIETY Daniel Freeman and
    Jason Freeman
THE APOCRYPHAL GOSPELS
    Paul Foster
ARCHAEOLOGY Paul Bahn
ARCHITECTURE Andrew Ballantyne
ARISTOCRACY William Doyle
ARISTOTLE Jonathan Barnes
ART HISTORY Dana Arnold
ART THEORY Cynthia Freeland
ASTROBIOLOGY David C. Catling
ASTROPHYSICS James Binney
ATHEISM Julian Baggini
AUGUSTINE Henry Chadwick
AUSTRALIA Kenneth Morgan

Available soon:

For more information visit our website

www.oup.com/vsi/

Les Iversen

DRUGS

A Very Short Introduction

SECOND EDITION

OXFORD
UNIVERSITY PRESS

Great Clarendon Street, Oxford, OX2 6DP,
United Kingdom

Oxford University Press is a department of the University of Oxford.
It furthers the University's objective of excellence in research, scholarship,
and education by publishing worldwide. Oxford is a registered trade mark of
Oxford University Press in the UK and in certain other countries

First edition published in 2001
Second edition published in 2016

Impression: 1

Published in the United States of America by Oxford University Press
198 Madison Avenue, New York, NY 10016, United States of America

British Library Cataloguing in Publication Data

Data available

Library of Congress Control Number: 2015959273

ISBN 978-0-19-874579-2

Printed in Great Britain by
Ashford Colour Press Ltd, Gosport, Hampshire

Contents

List of illustrations

Chapter 1
History

The word 'drug' refers to a chemical substance that is taken
deliberately in order to obtain some desirable effect. Some drugs
are used medically to treat illnesses whereas others are taken
because of their pleasurable effects. Both uses are ancient in their
origins. The first humans were hunter-gatherers; they had to learn
which of the thousands of plants in their environment were good
to eat and which were poisonous. By trial and error they also
gradually accumulated knowledge of which plants or other natural
materials might help to relieve pain or treat the symptoms of their
illnesses. The consumption of medicinal plants is not restricted to
humans, studies of chimpanzee behaviour have revealed that sick
animals sometimes select plants not usually contained in their
diet for their antiparasitic effects.

Humans at first did not accept death as a natural phenomenon.
Serious diseases were believed to be of supernatural origin: the
work of an enemy, visitation by a malevolent demon, or the work
of an offended god who had stolen the victim's soul. The treatment
was intended to lure the errant soul back to its proper habitat
within the body by counterspells, incantations, potions, suction, or
other means. On the other hand minor ailments such as colds or
constipation were accepted as part of existence and dealt with by
means of such herbal remedies as were available. Before there was
a written language, knowledge of plant medicines was handed on

1

by word of mouth from one generation to another. This eventually became a specialized occupation for the 'medicine man', 'shaman', or 'witch doctor', who often combined medical knowledge with the practice of magic and religious rites and became a potent and powerful figure in the community. The belief in spirits that could interfere with life for good or evil, and therefore could cause disease, was almost universal, so it is not surprising that knowledge of drugs was combined with this superstitious role.

Herbal pharmacopoeias

Among the earliest written records of herbal medicines are those from ancient China. The earliest book was the *Shen-Nung Pen T'sao Ching*, published during the Han dynasty in the 2nd century CE; it listed 365 herbal medicines and became an important basis for the development of Chinese medicine. The book was added to many times. A particularly important revision, *Pen T'sao Keng Mu* (the 'Great Pharmacopoeia'), prepared by Li Shin Chen during the Ming dynasty in the 16th century, was in fifty-two volumes and listed 1,898 medicines of plant, animal, and mineral origins. Li was one of the first to study drugs scientifically; he personally studied the actions of many traditional remedies. As a result he discarded a lot of useless information and eliminated some toxic preparations. Pharmacology is the scientific study of drugs, so Li could perhaps be called the first pharmacologist. He also compiled one of the first pharmacopoeias: a book containing directions for the identification of compound medicines.

Herbal medicines continue to be important in modern Chinese medicine, and many active substances have been introduced into Western medicine from these sources. In traditional Chinese medicine various preparations are mixed in complex prescriptions according to philosophical principles, to restore the harmony of the yin and the yang and the balance between the five organs, the five planets, and the five colours. The art of prescribing these Chinese remedies is complex, and is very different from the use of drugs in modern Western medicine, in which single pure chemical substances are used to treat particular aspects of illness.

In India, the ancient ayurvedic system of medicine originated as long as 3,000 years ago. It remains widely practised in Asia, and it too relies heavily on natural drugs, often in complex mixtures. Unlike the relatively benign and non-toxic effects of most Chinese medicines, however, the ayurvedic approach often seems to be more aggressive—with drug-induced vomiting, purging of the gut with laxatives and enemas, and bleeding as common remedies. A number of medical texts also exist from ancient Egypt (2000–1500 BCE), describing the use of many herbal and natural medicines: senna, honey, thyme, juniper, frankincense, cumin and colocynth (for digestion); pomegranate root and henbane (for worms); and also flax, oakgall, pine-tar, manna, bayberry, acanthus, aloe, caraway, cedar, coriander, cypress, elderberry, fennel, garlic, wild lettuce, nasturtium, onion, papyrus, poppy plant, saffron, sycamore, and watermelon.

Systemized herbal pharmacopoeias also emerged independently in other cultures. The father of modern medicine, Hippocrates, founded one of the first schools of 'rational' or 'scientific' medicine, and used several hundred natural medicines. In Greece Dioscorides published his influential *De material medica* in CE 55, and this was considered an absolute authority for the next 1,600 years. In ancient Rome Pliny (CE 60) published his *Natural History*, the largest ever compilation of knowledge of herbal and other natural remedies. Herbal medicine flourished elsewhere too, notably in the medieval era in the Arab world and in Europe. The British herbal pharmacopoeia written by Nicholas Culpeper (1616–54) was one of the most famous; he combined herbal remedies with astrology. An example of the many medical uses of comfrey advocated by Culpeper is shown in Box 1.

The era of herbal medicine lasted for many centuries. Herbal remedies included several very potent and effective medicines, but

Box 1 Culpepper on comfrey

'The roots of Comfrey taken fresh, beaten small and spread upon leather, and laid upon any place troubled with the gout, does presently give ease of the pains; and applied in the same manner, giveth ease to pained joints, and profiteth very much for running and moist ulcers, gangrenes, mortifications, and the like, for which it hath often experience been found helpful.'

Culpeper 1659

there was also much mythology. According to the 'Doctrine of Signatures', remedies for disease could be recognized by some property or 'signature' that they possessed. For example, lungwort (Pulmonaria), which resembles the tissue inside the lungs, was used for a variety of respiratory ailments; saffron because of its yellow colour was used to treat jaundice; and the mandrake plant and ginseng were used for many ailments because their roots often resembled the human form.

The era of scientific medicine

The Renaissance saw the development of a new experimental approach to medicine in the great medical schools of Europe, and the rediscovery of medical knowledge from ancient Greece and Rome. But it was not until the 19th century that scientific medicine really began to have a major impact on the practice of medicine. A key discovery was that infectious diseases were caused by microscopic living organisms. The main credit for this is due to the French chemist Louis Pasteur. It was Pasteur who, by a brilliant series of experiments, proved that the fermentation of wine and the souring of milk are caused by living microorganisms. His work led to the pasteurization of milk and solved problems of agriculture and industry as well as those of animal and human diseases. He successfully employed inoculations (vaccines) to prevent anthrax in sheep and cattle, chicken cholera in fowl, and finally rabies in humans and dogs.

From Pasteur, Joseph Lister derived the concepts that enabled him to introduce the antiseptic principle into surgery. Up until the mid-century surgical operations and childbirth were associated with a high risk of infection and often death. In 1865 Lister, a professor of surgery at Glasgow University, began placing an antiseptic barrier of carbolic acid between the wound and the germ-containing atmosphere. Infections and deaths fell dramatically, and his pioneering work led to more refined techniques of sterilizing the surgical environment.

The first anaesthetic, nitrous oxide ('laughing gas'), was described by Humphrey Davy in 1799, and is still used today in dental anaesthesia. William Morton, an American dentist, made surgical operations and childbirth less terrifying by the introduction of ether as an anaesthetic in 1846. Another major advance in surgery came from Edinburgh, where the Professor of Midwifery, James Young Simpson, had been experimenting upon himself and his assistants, inhaling various vapours with the object of discovering an effective anaesthetic. In November 1847 chloroform was tried with complete success, and it soon became the anaesthetic of choice. In Britain, official royal sanction was given to anaesthetics by Queen Victoria, who accepted chloroform from her physician, John Snow, when giving birth to her eighth child, Prince Leopold, in 1853.

It was in 19th-century Germany, however, that the development of the modern era of drug development began. Germany was a leader in the scientific approach to medicine, and students flocked to German medical schools from all over the world. German chemists were the first to isolate pure drug chemicals from herbal medicines, with the isolation of morphine from crude opium in 1803 and quinine from the bark of the cinchona tree in 1820. Morphine was used as a powerful pain reliever, but, like opium before it, morphine also became a drug of abuse. Quinine had a major impact on the prevention and treatment of malaria. One of the outstanding scientific leaders of that era was Paul Ehrlich. While still a student, Ehrlich carried out work on lead poisoning from which he evolved the theory that was to guide much of his subsequent work—that certain tissues have a selective affinity for certain chemicals. This led in turn to the modern concept that drugs are recognized by specific receptors in the body (see Chapter 2), and indeed Ehrlich was one of the first to use the term 'receptor'. In the early 20th century J. N. Langley, Professor of Physiology in Cambridge, England, studied the actions of nicotine and the South American arrow poison curare on nerve-muscle preparations, and also concluded that the drugs act on a 'receptive substance' that is neither nerve nor muscle.

The last half of the 20th century and the early years of the 21st saw an unprecedented flourishing of basic medical research and a remarkable increase in the kinds and numbers of drugs available for clinical use. The list of disease conditions that could be treated expanded enormously, and the discovery and production of new synthetic drugs for sale became a major industry. The top-selling drugs nowadays are mainly biologics, proteins, or antibodies, made on biological templates rather than chemically synthesized. Annual sales of medical drugs in the USA increased from $149 million in 1939 to a staggering $1057.2 billion in 2014—an increase of more than a thousandfold. The impact that these new medicines have had on human life and well-being has been extraordinary.

Our love affair with recreational drugs

As a species we have a unique propensity to seek out mind-altering chemicals and sometimes to persist in their use even when we know that such behaviour may be damaging to our health. Animals also seem to enjoy intoxicants. For example, apes in the wild will get mildly drunk on over-ripe fruit that has fermented to produce alcohol. My cats enjoy their Christmas treat of a small cloth mouse stuffed with the dried leaves of catmint (Nepeta); they roll wildly on the floor chewing fiercely on this toy and inhaling the intoxicating vapours. But apes do not allow the search for over-ripe fruit to dominate their lives, and my cats do not seek out a regular supply of catmint, even though it is available in our garden.

The recreational use of drugs seems to have been a part of human behaviour for many thousands of years. Alcohol was probably the first such drug—it is easily available from fruit and wild yeasts that are common in most parts of the world. It was a small step to discover how to control the process of fermentation to make wines and beer. There are records of organized drinking houses in ancient Babylon more than 3,000 years ago, and wine making was common in all parts of the Roman Empire. Alcoholic beverages appear in the Hebrew Bible, after Noah planted a vineyard and became inebriated. The production of alcoholic drinks in their almost infinite variety has become a large industry, and their consumption, except in Islamic countries, is widespread around the world. Like many other recreational drugs, alcohol has also been widely used in medicine—as a rough and ready anaesthetic in the era before ether and chloroform, and as an ingredient in many patent medicines—including gripe water (a dilute sugary alcoholic drink) for restless babies with colic, although nowadays gripe water no longer contains alcohol. Alcohol also plays a role in various religions, as in the communion wine of Christianity. The excessive use of alcohol and the liability to dependence came into special prominence in the deprived cities of the industrial era of the 19th and 20th centuries, where gin was cheap. Most countries reacted by placing restrictive laws on the sale of alcohol and by taxing it heavily. During World War I, claims that war production was being hampered by drunkenness led to pub opening times being restricted and alcohol strength reduced (Defence of the Realm Act, 1914). Despite this, the past twenty years saw the emergence of 'binge drinking'—people drinking enough alcohol in one session to end up in a stupor.

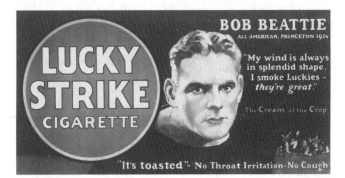

1. In the 1920s advertisements for cigarettes conveyed a healthy message.

Smoking tobacco in its various forms was for more than fifty years the most popular form of recreational drug use in the Western world in the 20th century (see Figure 1). The tobacco plant *Nicotiana rustica* is native to North America, and smoking the dried leaves was a custom among many of the American Indian tribes. Smoking formed an important part of Indian ceremonies, such as the smoking of the pipe of peace, and they also believed that tobacco possessed medicinal properties. Christopher Columbus brought the plant and the habit to Europe and it spread rapidly. The early European colonists in America grew tobacco for export to Europe, and it rapidly became the chief commodity of their trade. In 1604, King James I of England published an anti-smoking treatise, *A Counterblaste to Tobacco*, that had the effect of raising taxes on tobacco.

In India and in the Arab world, smoking the burning leaves of another plant, *Cannabis sativa*, has been widely practised for thousands of years. The dried leaves ('marijuana'), and the more potent female flowering heads of the plant ('sinsemilla'), or the sticky cannabis resin, can be smoked or consumed in a variety of foodstuffs. In the Hindu religion cannabis plays an important ritual role, and in Islamic countries, where the use of alcohol is

8

forbidden, cannabis use—which is not explicitly mentioned in the Koran—has sometimes taken its place. The use of cannabis as a recreational drug was virtually unknown in the West until the mid-20th century, when it became popular with the beat and hippie generation of the 1960s and 1970s. Since then it has become firmly embedded in Western culture, as the third most widely consumed recreational drug after alcohol and tobacco. Plant-breeders in California and in Holland have developed new strains of cannabis plant with an enhanced content of the active ingredient, Δ^9-tetrahydrocannabinol (THC). Apart from its intoxicant effects, cannabis also has a number of potentially important medicinal uses, and has been widely used in Indian medicine for many centuries. It was also used in Western medicine for almost one hundred years from the mid-19th until the mid-20th century.

The coca leaf was not burned but chewed by Peruvian Indians and was regarded by the Incas as a symbol of divinity. The Spanish conquistadores, however, regarded coca chewing as a vice, and, unlike tobacco, this habit was never introduced into European society. When the active ingredient cocaine was isolated as a pure chemical by the German chemist Albert Niemann in 1860, however, the drug suddenly became popular because of its medicinal properties. It was the first effective local anaesthetic to be used in delicate surgery on the eye and in dentistry. For a decade or more cocaine was used for a variety of medical conditions, and was famously championed by Sigmund Freud. Cocaine was said to be effective in treating a variety of nervous complaints and also began to be used recreationally. The original Coca-Cola® contained cocaine as an infusion of coca leaves, and a range of 'coca wine' preparations became available as patent medicines (see Figure 2); lozenges containing cocaine were even marketed by the E. Merck Company to impart a 'silvery quality' to the singing voice. Ironically, one of the medical uses was in the treatment of opium addiction—a condition that was beginning to be recognized in the late 19th century. The powerful addictive

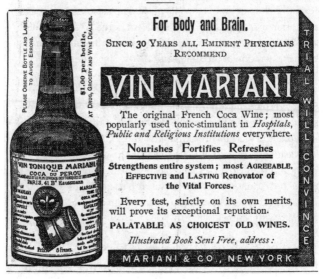

Drugs

2. Cocaine-containing medicines were freely sold in the early 20th century as remedies for a variety of ills. This advert promotes one of the many different coca wines that were recommended as 'tonic-stimulants'.

properties of cocaine soon became apparent, however, and both medical and non-medical use fell almost completely out of favour until the modern revival of cocaine as a recreational drug in the late 20th century.

Opium, the dried resin of the poppy plant, is another example of an ancient medicine that also served recreational purposes throughout history. Opium is one of the oldest effective painkillers, and figures prominently in both Eastern and Western herbal medicine. In Britain opium was imported in large quantities throughout the 19th century and enjoyed unrestricted medical and non-medical use (see Box 2). The impoverished labourer could buy a sample of raw opium from the corner shop

Box 2 Opium in 19th-century Britain

'The opium preparations on sale and stocked by chemist's shops were numerous. There were opium pills (or soap and opium, and lead and opium pills), opiate lozenges, compound powder of opium, opiate confection, opiate plaster, opium enema, opium linament, vinegar of opium and wine of opium. There was a famous tincture of opium (opium dissolved in alcohol), known as laudanum, which had widespread popular sale, and the camphorated tincture, or paregoric. The dried capsules of the poppy were used, as were poppy fomentation, syrup of white poppy and extract of poppy. There were nationally famous and long established preparations like Dover's Powder, that mixture of ipecacuanha and powdered opium originally prescribed for gout by Dr Thomas Dover. . . . An expanding variety of commercial preparations began to come on the market at mid-century. They were typified by the chlorodynes—Collis Browne's, Towle's and Freeman's. The children's opiates like Godfrey's Cordial and Dalby's Carminative were long established [and used by working mothers to keep their children quiet while they went out to work]. They were everywhere to be bought. There were local preparations, too, like Kendal Black Drop, popularly supposed to be four times the strength of laudanum—and well known outside its locality because Coleridge used it. Poppy head tea in the Fens, 'sleepy beer' in the Crickhowell area, Nepenthe, Owbridge's Lung Tonic, Battley's sedative solution—popular remedies, patent medicines and the opium preparations of the textbooks were all available.'

Berridge and Edwards, *Opium and the People*, p. 24

and enjoy an evening of oblivion; the children of working-class families could be dosed the opium-containing 'cordials' to keep them quiet while the parents went to work; the children sometimes died. The middle-class matron would use the more refined laudanum—an alcoholic extract of opium, diluted in water and consumed to while away the dull afternoons. Opium was an important product in the economy of the British Empire, and Britain used the political weapon of the 'Opium Wars' with China (1839–60) to force the Chinese to accept the importation of opium from India. Opium, and later the pure compound morphine, formed the base for hundreds of different medicines. Opium consumption rose to new heights in the latter part of the 19th century, and the invention of the hypodermic syringe in 1850 allowed morphine and the more powerful synthetic derivative heroin to be administered directly into the bloodstream. There were no restrictions on opium use in England until 1868, when the first Pharmacy Act became law. It was only then that addiction was recognized as a problem on both sides of the Atlantic. By 1900 it was estimated that one in 500 of the US population was addicted to opium and strict regulation of supply soon followed—with only mixed success.

The 20th century saw the first entirely synthetic drugs that alter consciousness. The first of these were the amphetamines. d-Amphetamine (dexedrine) was first synthesized in the early 20th century and used because of its ability to constrict blood vessels. Sold as 'Benzedrine' and administered by drops or inhaler, it helped to ease nasal congestion. During World War II, dexedrine took on a new role as a stimulant that was used to keep military personnel alert and awake for long periods—for example, bomber crews on long flying missions. More potent forms of amphetamine, for example, methamphetamine ('speed'), and new forms of administering this drug by smoking continue to be widely abused. At the same time, the synthetic sedatives paraldehyde and chloral became available.

Throughout history the medical and non-medical uses of drugs have been closely interrelated. Thus, morphine has always been one of the most important drugs in the pharmacopoeia—but also one of the most dangerous drugs of abuse (see Chapter 4). In the

Box 3 The discovery of d-LSD

The Swiss chemist Albert Hoffmann first synthesized d-lysergic acid diethylamide (d-LSD) in 1938 as one of a series of chemicals related to ergotamine, a drug isolated from a fungus that sometimes grew on crops of rye. Five years later he synthesized the compound again, and unwittingly received a minute dose of this powerful hallucinogen—perhaps through his skin. He describes what happened next:

'How dull would life be, if one of its dominating factors, what we call accident or chance were missing, and if we would never become surprised. I was very surprised, when in the afternoon of 16 April 1943, after I had repeated the synthesis of LSD, I entered suddenly into a kind of dream world. The surroundings had changed in a strange way, and had become luminous, more expressive. I felt uneasy and went home, where I wanted to rest. Lying on the couch with closed eyes, because I experienced daylight as unpleasantly glaring, I perceived an uninterrupted stream of fantastic pictures, with an intense kaleidoscopic play of colors. After some hours this strange but not unpleasant condition faded away.'

Hoffmann (1994)

early years of the new millennium the medical use of cannabis has been reintroduced in several European countries, and in many states in the USA.

The story of the accidental discovery of d-LSD is another example of the synthesis of a powerful mind-altering chemical (see Box 3). The discovery of LSD prompted the rediscovery of other plant-derived hallucinogens—mescaline from cactus, and psilocybin from the Mexican 'magic mushroom' teonanactl. Both had featured prominently in ancient religious rites.

During the past hundred years there have been dramatic increases in both the medical and the recreational use of drugs. In the medical field breakthroughs occurred in our ability to control life-threatening illnesses, and for the first time drugs allowed us to take control of our own reproduction. The increased use of recreational drugs occurred in response both to poverty and deprivation in some communities, and to affluence in others. Supplying and marketing both legal and illegal drugs became a major worldwide industry, accounting for a significant proportion of all economic activity.

Chapter 2
How drugs work

Drugs are chemicals: a series of atoms bonded together to form a molecule. They can be of natural origin—extracted from plants, animals, or microbes. For example, many antibiotics used in the treatment of infectious diseases are chemicals synthesized by one micro-organism to protect itself against others. The powerful anti-cancer drug taxol is extracted from the leaves of the yew tree. Most drugs are man-made chemicals designed to act on some particular biochemical target, In the 21st century, however, there are an increasing number of 'biologicals'—proteins and antibodies made on a biological template. These are composed of chains of amino acids and are substantially larger molecules. Synthetic drugs are usually relatively small molecules, containing 10–100 atoms. Larger biological molecules, such as proteins (2,000–20,000 atoms), are not easily absorbed into the body and tend to be rapidly degraded on entry into the digestive system. They need to be administered directly by injection. Medicines contain the active drug molecule along with various other inactive ingredients, sugars, starches, or oils to make a tablet or other preparation. The amount of active drug is usually minute, measured in a few thousandths of a gram; it would be impractical to handle and manufacture tablets unless they contained some inert 'filler'.

Most medicines are taken by mouth in tablet or capsule form, but some are given as liquids (easier for children or old people to swallow), or by other routes of delivery, including injection. When medicines are given by mouth, they are gradually absorbed into the bloodstream from the stomach and gut. This is a relatively slow process—but this is not a drawback if the medicine is being used to treat a long-term disease, where a sustained delivery of drug is needed. The ideal medicine for such diseases is taken by mouth once a day—but this requires that there is a steady absorption from the gut and that the active drug is not degraded too rapidly in the body. Absorption from the gut need not involve swallowing the drug—another method is to administer the drug incorporated into a waxy suppository inserted into the rectum. This too gives a slow and sustained absorption of the active material and is a popular method of drug delivery in several European countries. When my wife developed a sore throat in Paris some years ago and went to a pharmacy to obtain some medicine she emerged with some strange-looking waxy lozenges, which she was about to swallow before our friends told her the correct means of administration! In Anglo-Saxon countries we are more prudish, and the rectal suppository has never been popular.

Some drugs require more rapid delivery—for example, an antibiotic given to treat a severe infection or an anaesthetic administered for a surgical operation. In such cases a drug solution can be injected directly into the blood via a vein. Intravenous injection is also a route favoured by drug addicts to deliver, for example, heroin—this route provides almost instant delivery of the drug to the brain, giving the maximum 'high'. Most biologicals are unstable in the gut and thus cannot be delivered by mouth and must be given by injection—often into muscle or just under the skin, or intravenously directly into the bloodstream.

Some recreational drug-users and addicts use smoking as a means of rapid delivery of drugs such as nicotine (tobacco smoke), cannabis, cocaine, or heroin. Many drugs are rapidly absorbed into the blood vessels present in the large internal surface area of

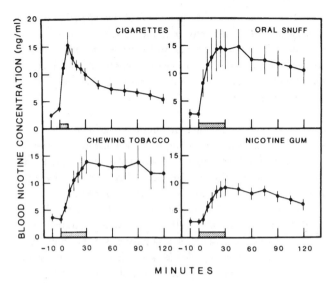

3. Absorption of nicotine via different routes. Drugs are absorbed into the bloodstream at different rates according to the route of administration. In the case of nicotine, smoking is the fastest means of delivering the drug, which is rapidly absorbed by the large surface area of the lungs.

the lungs (see Figure 3). The cigarette-smoker can obtain a pulse of nicotine to the brain within seconds of lighting up—and can then adjust the delivery of nicotine very precisely by controlling the frequency of puffs and the depth of inhalation. Because of the rapid delivery offered by this route, many anaesthetics are delivered by inhalation; as with the cigarette-smoker, the anaesthetist can control the level of anaesthesia very precisely by varying the rate of drug delivery. Some drugs are delivered locally to the site in the body at which they are needed—thus avoiding exposure of the whole body to what might be an undesirably large dose of the drug. For example, an aerosol of drug-containing fluid droplets is inhaled into the lung to control the symptoms of asthma; ointments are rubbed into the skin for pain relief; or medicines are given directly to the eye in the form of drops. Drugs used to treat disorders of the brain have to have special properties because the brain is insulated from the bloodstream by a specialized 'blood–brain barrier', which protects the brain from the possibly harmful effects of chemicals absorbed in the diet. Only small and relatively fat-soluble drug molecules are able to penetrate this barrier.

There have been several modern improvements in drug delivery systems. Special tablets can be designed that dissolve only slowly in the gut—providing an extended period of drug absorption. In this way it has been possible, for example, to develop a once-a-day preparation of morphine for pain relief—a considerable achievement for a drug that is inactivated quite rapidly and normally has to be given every four hours. Another advance has been the development of adhesive skin patches that contain an active drug and allow its prolonged absorption through the skin. This, for example, is a widely used means of delivering oestrogen as hormone replacement therapy for post-menopausal women.

Drug receptors

Whatever route of delivery is used, either the drug molecule must end up in the bloodstream—from which it can exit freely into virtually any organ of the body (apart from the brain)—or the drug must be delivered locally to the target organ. In the target organ, the drug is recognized by 'receptors'. These are large molecules, usually proteins, to which the drug binds tightly and with a high degree of specificity. Small changes in the chemistry of the drug molecule may yield analogues that are unable to bind and are consequently inactive. The drug often binds to a site in the protein normally occupied by some naturally occurring substance. Occupation of this site by the drug molecule then either mimics the effect normally elicited by that natural chemical (for drugs known as 'agonists') or blocks it ('antagonists'). For example, there are so-called beta-receptors in the heart, which recognize the cardiac stimulant hormone epinephrine (adrenaline). Epinephrine itself (the agonist) can be used in medical emergencies to stimulate the failing heart, but synthetic drugs called beta-blockers, which act as antagonists at the cardiac beta-receptors, are also valuable medicines, which are used to treat heart disease and high blood pressure (see Chapter 3). Drug molecules often exist in (d-) and (l-) mirror image forms known as enantiomers, new drugs increasingly use only the most active enantiomer in the final product.

Many drugs act on receptor protein molecules that normally function in cell signalling mechanisms. These proteins are located at the cell surface in various tissues (muscle, nerve, gut, brain, and so on). They may recognize and be activated by hormones carried in the bloodstream. For example, adrenaline (epinephrine) is secreted into the blood at times of stress and prepares the body for 'fight or flight'. It acts as a trigger for receptors present in many different parts of the body. Adrenaline stimulates the heart to pump more blood, mobilizes energy reserves in muscle, increases the rate of breathing, and in animals with fur it causes the individual hairs to rise—making the animal look bigger and more ferocious. Receptors on nerve cells recognize and respond to the many other different chemical messenger molecules used for communication between such cells in the brain. The binding of the natural signal molecule activates such receptor proteins. This leads to a subtle change in the shape of the protein, which may trigger changes in the permeability of the cell to sodium, potassium, calcium, or other inorganic ions, thus altering its excitability. Alternatively, the activated receptor may trigger the synthesis of other internal signalling molecules within the cell, the so-called 'second messengers' that alter the cell's metabolism. Several hundred such cell surface receptor proteins are known—and more are being discovered, as we understand more about the human genome. A typical receptor protein consists of 400–500 amino-acid residues. Many are folded and inserted into the cell membrane in such a way that there are seven regions of the protein within the membrane and some regions protruding on

19

both external and internal surfaces. Detailed knowledge of the molecular architecture of such receptors is helping us to understand better how they work, and in future may help in the design of drug molecules to fit the receptor even more precisely. Many drugs activate the receptor site normally activated by the natural agonist, or act as antagonists by competing with the natural agonist at its binding site and preventing its normal action. Recently another category of drugs has been found, which change the sensitivity of a receptor to its normal agonist, but which bind at a site other than that where the natural agonist binds. Such 'allosteric' drugs can up-regulate or down-regulate receptor function.

Other proteins located at the surface of the cell can also be drug targets. A large family of proteins function as gatekeepers, regulating the levels of chemicals in the cell, particularly the components of the salty solution in which all living cells are bathed. These include sodium, potassium, calcium, chloride, and other inorganic salts. The gatekeeper proteins form minute channels in the cell membrane through which such chemicals can enter or exit living cells—and by changes in the protein's shape these channels can be opened or closed according to need. Such channels are particularly important in nerve cells and in muscle, which rely on an imbalance between salts inside and outside the cell to generate the minute pulses of electricity by which nerve signals are transmitted or which cause muscles to contract. These channels offer a rich variety of drug targets. The ancient remedy digitalis, extracted from the foxglove plant, for example, acts by blocking sodium channels in heart muscle, preventing potentially dangerous overactivity. Other cell surface proteins act as 'pumps' that transport chemicals from one side of the cell membrane to the other—usually from the outside to the inside. They have a number of functions—for example, in delivering glucose or other nutrients to the cell, or in removing biologically active chemicals from the cell surface. The antidepressant drug Prozac, for example, acts by blocking a pump whose function is to remove the chemical messenger molecule serotonin after its release from activated nerve cells. Blocking this pump has the effect of prolonging the actions of serotonin in the brain—and this appears to underlie its antidepressant properties (see Chapter 3).

Drugs may act on biochemical targets within the cell as well as at the cell surface. Some drugs bind directly to DNA in the nucleus and interfere with the normal process of reading DNA sequences into proteins, thereby inhibiting cell division and growth. This can be particularly important in some drugs used to control the growth of cancer cells. Other targets inside the cell include enzymes. Enzymes are proteins that have the special function of acting as catalysts to promote particular chemical reactions that are involved in the breakdown of foodstuffs to produce energy, or in the synthesis of one or other of the complex chemicals that make up the body. Such chemical syntheses often involve a complex series of reactions and a number of different enzymes. Blocking the action of one enzyme with a drug can, however, block the whole pathway. This strategy has yielded many very important medical drugs. For example, many antibiotics act by blocking the synthesis of key components of the bacterial cell wall, thus preventing further bacterial multiplication; cholesterol-lowering drugs inhibit an enzyme involved in cholesterol synthesis. Enzyme proteins contain an 'active site' that normally binds the chemical substrate of the enzyme. Inhibitor drugs usually bind to the same site and prevent the enzyme from functioning. Enzymes are often soluble proteins present in the cell sap within living cells. For technical reasons, this makes it easier to obtain precise information on their three-dimensional molecular structure—and this in turn assists in the application of computer-aided molecular modelling techniques to design drugs that target that particular enzyme and 'dock' into its active site.

The science of genetics, which aims to study how individual characteristics are inherited, advanced greatly during the last twenty years. This was largely due to powerful new technology that allowed scientists to characterize DNA molecules. These long thread-like molecules in the nucleus of every cell in the body carry the information needed to specify proteins, encoded in the sequence of the four bases of which they are composed—adenine, thymine, cytosine, and guanine. The DNA for an individual gene consists of a sequence of several thousand bases that specifies the sequence of the twenty different amino-acid building blocks that are linked together to form a protein, containing on average 500–1,000 amino acids. The 'human genome' project was an international effort; it cost more than $100 million and took thirteen years to successfully sequence the entire human DNA sequence of more than three billion bases, encoding some 30,000 different genes, and was a landmark achievement. DNA sequencing methods have since improved radically, so that a single human genome can now be sequenced in a matter of days, at a cost of around $1,000. We will soon be able to purchase a read-out of our own unique genome. This offers the hope that particular gene sequences may be related to particular human diseases, opening a new era of individually tailored medicines. Massive research efforts are now devoted to this goal (see Chapter 6).

Meanwhile it is now possible to isolate the human DNA encoding for a particular protein and to insert this into a tissue culture cell. The resulting newly created cells, sometimes described as 'immortal', will grow and divide indefinitely, and will express the protein of interest. Molecular pharmacologists can thus study human drug receptors under laboratory conditions—and can use these model systems to discover new drugs that target that particular receptor. The profile of activity of new drugs can be determined with a minute amount of the drug tested simultaneously against fifty or more drug targets using automated laboratory robots. This technology can be applied both to cell surface receptor proteins and to enzymes. For enzymes it is also possible to insert the human gene into a bacterium, which will then make the human enzyme. It is usually easy to grow large quantities of bacteria, so in this way it is possible to produce large amounts of human enzyme protein that can later be extracted and purified. Enzyme proteins that may be present normally only in minute amounts in the body can thus be produced in large quantities for laboratory studies and for use in screening new drugs. The new era of molecular pharmacology allows a scientist to study human drug receptors in a way that was not possible before. Previous studies of drug receptors have relied on using indirect tests of receptor function—in which the receptor was a 'black box' of unknown biochemical composition. Prior to the molecular pharmacology era, studying the actions of drugs on receptors usually involved using receptors in the tissues of laboratory animals. Although human drug receptors and those found in laboratory animals (e.g. rats and mice) are usually very similar, there can be important species differences.

Measuring the effects of drugs

Although molecular techniques can tell us a great deal about the way in which drug molecules interact with their receptors, other methods are needed to assess the effects of drugs in the body. Some of the biological effects of drugs can be studied in human or animal cells grown in tissue culture in the laboratory. Thus, the actions of drugs on the electrical activity of brain cells can be examined by using minute needle-like electrodes to record such activity directly from individual nerve cells growing in tissue culture. Alternatively, heart muscle cells in tissue culture can be used to examine the effects of drugs on the excitability of the heart. The effectiveness of new antibiotics in killing bacteria or other microorganisms can also readily be assessed in the test tube or Petri dish. A whole era of pharmacology relied on the use of isolated animal organs after removal from the body (for example, heart, muscle, segments of gut), which continue to contract for some time after removal if incubated in oxygenated warm saline solution. Drugs can then be added to the 'organ bath' and their effects studied by measuring the resulting changes in muscle contraction or heartbeat.

Eventually, however, we want to know what effects drugs have on the whole organism. If we want to study the effects of drugs on blood pressure, we cannot expect to do this just by examining their effects on cells in tissue culture or on isolated organs; we need to measure blood pressure in human or animal subjects. If we are interested in testing new drugs to treat epileptic seizures, we need to use animal models in which epileptic seizures can be simulated by various means. In the final analysis, we need to give the drugs to human patients suffering from epilepsy to see if they are effective. However, it would be unethical to give new drugs of unknown toxicity to human subjects in the first instance, so animal experiments still inevitably play a crucial role in studying the effects of drugs. The advent of molecular techniques that allow the initial screening of new compounds to be carried out with human cells in the laboratory means that the numbers of animals needed for drug research has gone down markedly in recent years. A large range of different animal models exists for studying the effects of various categories of drugs. In cases where the medical end point is clearly defined and the biological mechanisms well understood—for example, in lowering blood pressure, reducing blood cholesterol, reducing inflammation, or fighting infectious diseases—the animal models can often provide a fairly precise replica of the human disease. In other illnesses, however, particularly in mental disorders, there is much less understanding of the biological basis of the illness. Animal models in these instances often involve complex behavioural tests, chosen because existing drugs that are known to be effective in these diseases have some clear effect.

Whatever test system is used, whether it is a simple biochemical measurement of drug/receptor binding in the test tube or the recording of a complex physiological or behavioural response in the whole animal, a key issue is to determine the effective drug dose. The drug concentration needed to occupy the receptor, and hence to produce a response, is determined by the affinity of the drug for the target receptor, i.e. the strength of the binding of the drug. If the affinity is high, only low concentrations of the drug will be needed, and only very low doses will be needed to elicit the desired response in the whole animal. To find out what the effective concentration is in the drug/receptor assay, or what dose is needed in the whole animal or person, a wide range of different drug concentrations or doses needs to be tested. The results can be presented as a graph showing the drug response with increasing doses—the so-called dose-response curve. As the range of effective drug concentrations often spans a range of more than a thousandfold, the drug concentration is usually depicted on a log scale (see Figure 4). The dose-response curve is useful, as it allows one to compare the potencies of a range of different drugs that act on the same receptor; a useful comparator is the drug concentration needed to produce a 50 per cent response (EC50). Although the actions of drugs reflect their ability to occupy their

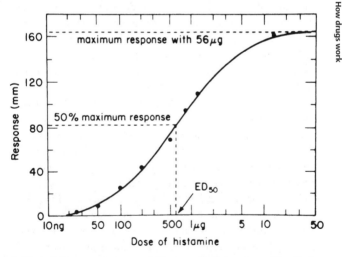

4. Typical 'dose-response curve'. Pharmacologists measure the effects of increasing doses of drug to find the maximum response and the 'effective dose 50' or 'ED50', which causes half of the maximum response. In this instance the contraction of a piece of guinea pig small intestine was measured in response to increasing doses of histamine.

particular receptor targets, the dose-response curve generated in the test tube or tissue culture model is not always reflected in the whole animal. When drugs are administered, they may not reach their desired targets, or they may be inactivated very rapidly. Drugs that target receptors in the brain may not be able to penetrate the blood–brain barrier. Thus, although the drug may have a high affinity for the right receptor, it may be quite inactive in the whole animal or person.

Finding the most suitable dose is one of the most difficult questions in using drugs to treat medical conditions. Virtually all drugs will produce undesirable side effects if too high a dose is given. These side effects can range from minor discomforts to life-threatening damage to vital organs—often gut, liver, or kidney. Even aspirin, a drug commonly believed to be safe, can cause dangerous irritation and bleeding in the stomach and intestine. Thousands of patients die each year from gastric bleeding caused by aspirin and the newer more powerful aspirin-like drugs. For most drugs there is an optimum range of doses that produces the maximum medical benefit without adverse side effects. The separation between the dose range in which the desirable medical benefits are seen, and the higher dose ranges at which adverse effects emerge, is known as the 'therapeutic window'. Obviously, it is desirable that this window should be as big as possible, but it is not always possible to achieve this. The adverse side effects may be caused by overstimulation of the same receptor mechanism that underlies the therapeutic effects. Thus, for example, morphine is widely used in treating severe pain, but the therapeutic window is relatively small and, at higher doses, nausea and vomiting, confusion, constipation and life-threatening respiratory depression are all common side effects, and these are all mediated by the same opiate receptor mechanism that mediates pain relief. Similarly, one of the problems encountered in the medical use of cannabis is that there is only a narrow therapeutic window between the doses that yield beneficial medical effects and the doses that cause intoxication. Although the intoxicant effects are what the recreational user wants from the drug, these effects are usually unwanted and can be frightening to the elderly patient not familiar with the drug. The therapeutic-window concept applies equally importantly to the recreational use of drugs. Even the experienced heroin or cocaine user sometimes gets it wrong and ends up taking a lethal overdose.

Finding the most suitable therapeutic dose for a new drug, and determining the size of the therapeutic window, are among the most difficult parts of any drug development. Because individual human beings differ in size and in the way in which they inactivate drug molecules, it may not be possible to define a dose that will be optimum for all patients, and it may be necessary to find this out by trial and error. The optimum dose may be different for men and women, who sometimes inactivate drugs differently; children and old people are also less able to inactivate drugs quickly, so they may need smaller doses than healthy adults.

How drugs are inactivated

As far as the body is concerned, drugs, whether natural or man-made, are foreign substances and a series of complex defences have evolved to inactivate and eliminate such materials. In the natural environment humans and other animals encounter a wide range of chemicals in their diet, many of which can have biological effects. It is clearly undesirable that such potentially dangerous chemicals should be allowed to accumulate—they must be detoxified and eliminated. Man-made drugs can also be inactivated and eliminated by these mechanisms, and this poses a problem for the pharmacologist. If the drug is inactivated and eliminated too rapidly, it will be effective for only a short period of time, and repeat dosing may be needed. In some instances—for example, in the use of morphine to control severe pain—the drug may need to be taken every few hours. The ideal for the long-term treatment of chronic illnesses is obviously a medicine that needs to be taken only once a day.

Some drugs will be excreted unchanged in the urine. The kidney has a number of specialized pump mechanisms that remove substances actively from the blood and pass them out in the urine—these mechanisms apply particularly to drugs that have some acidic or alkaline character that can be recognized by these kidney mechanisms. Fat-soluble drugs may be removed quite rapidly from the circulation, as they tend to become concentrated in fat stores in the body. Such drugs may persist for long periods in the fat stores and gradually leak out into circulation and become excreted. While dissolved in the fat, the drugs are not biologically active, as they do not have access to their receptors. Cannabis and some of its metabolites, for example, persist in the fat stores of the body for several weeks after a single dose. Because minute amounts leak out of the fat stores and are excreted in urine, the recreational user can yield a urine-positive cannabis drug test more than one week after a single exposure to the drug.

By far the most important means of inactivating drugs is by metabolism—using enzymes to convert them to harmless products, which can then be eliminated from the body. Much of this drug metabolism takes place in the liver, which is rich in a wide range of different drug-metabolizing enzymes. The liver is strategically placed. As it receives all of the blood coming from the gut before it enters the general circulation, it can eliminate toxic chemicals absorbed from the diet before they can do too much harm. Drug molecules are attacked by one or more of the liver enzymes and converted into inactive by-products that are then excreted, either in the bile from the liver, discharged into the gut and eventually eliminated in the faeces, or by the kidney into the urine. The drug-metabolizing enzymes in the liver, called cytochrome-p450s, comprise a large family of some fifty or more related enzymes, which have evolved in a remarkable way. They can deal with essentially any foreign chemical—including man-made drugs that by definition are never normally encountered in nature. Many drugs are given repeatedly for long periods of time and the liver and kidney are called upon every day

to eliminate these foreign chemicals. These organs are exposed
to high concentrations of drugs as they are first absorbed from
the gut and channelled through the liver, and the drug or its
metabolite may be concentrated in the kidney for excretion in the
urine. It is not surprising, therefore, that the liver and the kidney
are the organs that are most vulnerable to drug-induced damage.
This can sometimes be serious and even life threatening. The
metabolism of drugs in the liver can also sometimes produce
toxic metabolites that make matters worse, as in the case of the
relatively harmless drug paracetamol, which can be degraded
to form a liver-damaging metabolite.

One way of minimizing these risks is to develop and use more and
more potent drugs, so that the amount of foreign chemical that
needs to be given is reduced. In the older generation of medical
drugs it was not uncommon to need doses of 1 gram or more each
day, whereas with many modern drugs the doses needed are
100–1,000 times lower.

The efficiency of the various mechanisms for drug metabolism and
elimination poses a challenge to the pharmacologist, because these
processes limit the duration of action of drugs. Some drugs may be
well absorbed from the gut, but may suffer extensive metabolic
degradation in the liver before they have a chance to enter the
general circulation and exert their beneficial effects. An additional
problem that is often encountered is that different drugs may
compete for the same liver enzymes. In this case, their duration of
action and peak blood levels may be altered when given together,
often with adverse consequences. Such drug interactions are
common, particularly in elderly patients, who tend to be taking
several different medicines every day. Prolonged regimes of drug
treatment can cause another problem. If the same drug is taken
repeatedly, it may lead to a large increase in the liver enzyme(s)
involved in its metabolism; this means that the drug will tend to
become less and less effective over time—a phenomenon known as
'tolerance'. Drug interactions may also be seen in such instances: if

drug A leads to a large increase in liver enzyme activity, it may accelerate the disposal of drug B if this is metabolized by the same enzyme(s). Extracts of St John's wort have become popular as a natural antidepressant, for example, but it has become apparent that the herbal medicine causes increases in a number of liver enzymes and this can alter the effectiveness of several prescription drugs—notably the oral contraceptives and drugs used to treat AIDS.

We are also becoming increasingly aware of idiosyncratic responses of some people to drugs. This may be due to genetic factors that alter drug responsiveness in some individuals. For example, 6 per cent of the Caucasian population lacks the genes encoding one of the cytochrome p450 drug-metabolizing enzymes known as CYP2D6. This enzyme is importantly involved in the metabolism of about a quarter of all prescription drugs. Such individuals have a serious impairment in their ability to detoxify and eliminate these drugs and may thus overreact when treated with normal therapeutic doses. The study of genetic factors that determine drug responses is a new subject called 'pharmacogenomics'.

The inactivation of modern 'biological' medicines involves different mechanisms. Protein hormones (e.g. insulin, human growth hormone) are natural components in the circulation, and if administered as medicines they will be inactivated by the mechanisms used normally. Monoclonal antibodies, like naturally occurring antibodies, may circulate for long periods in the blood, and may thus not require frequent repeat dosing.

Some drugs, such as lithium, are not metabolized at all, but their rates of absorption and elimination are still important factors in determining their use.

Effects of long-term drug administration

Many drugs are used to treat chronic medical conditions and increasingly drugs are given prophylactically to prevent the development of a medical condition—as, for example, with the cholesterol-lowering agents (see Chapter 3). Such long-term dosage regimes may carry risks. As pointed out ('How drugs are inactivated', this chapter), it is not uncommon for the drugs to become less effective with time, because they cause an increase in liver-metabolizing enzymes. This is less likely to occur with modern highly potent drugs, as the increase in liver enzymes is usually seen only in response to relatively high doses of drugs, which swamp the liver's capacity to metabolize them. There are, however, other mechanisms that can lead to the development of drug tolerance. The use of morphine and related drugs as painkillers, for example, is complicated by the fact that most patients develop tolerance to the drug and require increasing doses—sometimes the drug becomes virtually ineffective even when given in very large doses. A tolerant patient can take as much as 1 gram of morphine a day—a dose that would prove lethal to a drug-naïve subject. In this case, the mechanisms responsible for the development of tolerance are not understood, but the phenomenon is nevertheless very real. Other drugs that act on the central nervous system also exhibit tolerance—and some also lead to the development of 'addiction' or 'substance dependence', as it is sometimes called (see Chapter 4). A special problem with the long-term administration of monoclonal antibodies is that they themselves cause an immune reaction. The early monoclonal antibodies were generated in mice without modification, and they rapidly caused immune reactions, which terminated their usefulness. Even the best humanized or fully human monoclonal antibodies may still prove to be immunogenic, and this may limit their long-term effectiveness.

Our understanding of how drugs work increased greatly during the 20th century. This ushered in an era of rational drug discovery, in which new drugs are made to target the particular biochemical mechanisms that are believed to be defective in individual diseases. The 21st century will see this approach extended, as we become able to design drugs that will best suit the individual patient.

Chapter 3
Drugs as medicines

The physician in the 21st century has an impressive range of powerful medicines at his or her command. It is possible to treat a number of hitherto untreatable conditions with effective medicines, and these often represent the most cost-effective way of managing illness by comparison with costly surgery or hospital care. Spending on drugs represents an average of around 10 per cent of the total health budget in most developed countries, and this will inevitably rise still further as an increasing number of expensive 'biologicals' becomes available. Medicines include the ever-popular herbal remedies, a variety of other natural products, and a host of man-made chemicals. A new generation of biological products is becoming increasingly important—they include human proteins that are used to replace their defective counterparts in some human diseases, and an increasing number of antibodies. These are proteins that are normally formed by the immune system as part of the body's defence against infections or invasion by other foreign bodies. The antibodies formed by the immune system in response to a vaccine will include some antibodies with high specificity for one or other of the proteins present in the vaccine challenge. These are made in minute amounts, however. The discovery that cells from the immune system could be merged with tumour cells to make the antibody-expressing cells capable of replication, made the manufacture of specific antibodies possible. The powerful techniques of molecular biology make it possible to synthesize such human antibodies and other human proteins on a large scale and to use them as medicines. More than 300 such monoclonal antibodies have been approved for medical use or are at earlier stages of development. The modern generation of monoclonal antibodies represents a new class of medicines, designed to target and inactivate various key proteins known to be involved in the processes underlying various diseases.

Most human proteins exist in only tiny amounts in the body, and hitherto the only way of obtaining them in any quantity was to purify them from blood or from human or animal tissues. By using the techniques of molecular biology a variety of human proteins can now be made, using their DNA template in tissue culture cells. For example, until recently most diabetic patients were treated with insulin purified from pig pancreas, but the synthetic human hormone now largely replaces this. Biological products are generally large proteins that cannot be absorbed when given by mouth—they have to be given by injection. Sometimes this may be needed several times a day (for example, insulin) but in other cases treatment once a week or once a month in the doctor's surgery may be sufficient.

Some medicines that are regarded as particularly safe to use can be obtained 'over-the-counter' in any pharmacy. These include such widely used drugs as the painkillers aspirin and paracetamol and a large number of medicines for coughs, colds, and other minor ailments. Such medicines are often based on traditional remedies and include a number of mildly active ingredients, together with sugars and flavouring to help make the medicine go down! Most new medical drugs, however, start life as prescription medicines. There is not enough experience of the possible hazards of a new medicine to make it safe to sell 'over-the-counter'. Doctors control the use of such medicines by writing a prescription and carefully monitoring the patient's response. If the drug is genuinely new, targeting a new mode of action with obvious clinical benefits, there will be an initial period during which the parent company enjoys a monopoly, and can charge a high price. This allows the company to make a profit and to regain the costs incurred in research and development of the new medicine. Other companies will soon copy the original drug, or its mechanism of action, and launch their own versions. In this phase competition will drive the price of these medicines down—but the original version will still enjoy the twenty years of monopoly offered by patent protection. Eventually, when patents expire, any drug manufacturer will be free to make and sell direct copies of the drug—a so-called generic version. This will cause the price of the drug to fall again—sometimes massively. At the end of this process, the innovative drug companies will have made considerable profits, and new medically important drugs will become available for mass use at low prices.

After many years of experience of the widespread use of a new prescription medicine, it may become clear that the compound is relatively safe to use—and it may then be sold 'over-the-counter'. In the 1990s, for example, a number of the powerful drugs used to treat stomach ulcers became available in this way—having first been available only as prescription drugs for nearly twenty years. On the other hand, with some drugs there will always be a risk to the patient if the dose is not right, or there may be the potential for diverting the medical drug to recreational use. It is unlikely, for example, that such drugs as antibiotics or opiate painkillers will be made into 'over-the-counter' products. Although morphine was available 'over-the-counter' in Victorian times, this is not likely to happen again.

This book is not intended to be a textbook of pharmacology—and in the space available it is impossible to cover the whole range of medical drugs now available. Instead a few examples will be highlighted to illustrate some of the principles underlying the successful use of medicines in the treatment of illnesses. Large omissions from this chapter include the drug treatment of blood diseases, diabetes, and other hormonal diseases.

Heart disease and high blood pressure

In 1628 William Harvey published his famous book *De motu cordis* in which he described the pumping action of the heart. Careful studies of various animals and human demonstrations led him to the then revolutionary idea that the blood circulated around the body, propelled by the heart acting as a pump. Hitherto it had been thought that the heart pumped air to cool the blood, aided by the lungs. We now know that the 4 litres or so of blood in an average human is pumped by the heart through the lungs for oxygenation and then via the arteries to all the tissues of the body, from which it is returned to the heart through the veins. The human heart has to perform prodigious mechanical feats—pumping the relatively viscous blood at quite high pressure through the millions of tiny capillary vessels in the tissues, and beating regularly for an entire lifetime. Its job is made more difficult in many people as they grow older because they develop abnormally high blood pressure. This is caused by the narrowing of blood vessels with age, making it more difficult for the heart to force the blood through them at normal pressure. These changes can be made worse by many different causes, of which obesity, too salty a diet, and smoking are some of the commonest. The high fat content of most Western diets tends to promote high blood levels of the insoluble fatty material cholesterol and this leads to the laying-down of deposits of cholesterol in the lining of the arteries. This in turn constricts the arteries and tends to lead to raised blood pressure. The cholesterol deposits are particularly dangerous when they affect the coronary arteries, the blood vessels within the heart muscle itself that supply it with oxygen and nutrients. The combination of raised blood pressure, which puts a greater burden on the heart as a pump, and partial blockade of the coronary arteries can lead to sudden heart failure, when one or more of the coronary vessels to the heart becomes entirely blocked. The patient will suffer sudden intense pain in the chest and arm. The outcome can be death, or recovery with a damaged heart, resulting in prolonged or permanent impairment. Coronary heart disease is one of the most common diseases and it remains one of the leading causes of death. Worldwide deaths from cardiovascular disease were estimated to be 17.5 million in 2012, representing 31 per cent of all deaths. In the USA 1 in 4 of all deaths were caused by cardiovascular disease, some 610,000 in total. High blood pressure and constricted arteries to the brain can also lead to stroke—a sudden interruption of the blood supply to vital areas of the brain. This too can lead to death or serious disability. Nevertheless, the advent of powerful new medicines is beginning to improve these statistics. Such improvements will continue during the initial decades of the 21st century, as the new treatments begin to show their long-term beneficial effects. The successful treatment of high blood pressure, heart disease, and abnormally high cholesterol were major achievements for pharmacology in the latter half of the 20th century.

The drugs used to treat high blood pressure come in many different varieties. Among the earliest to be developed were 'water pills' (diuretics), which promote urine production in the kidney. By removing some of the water content of the blood the drugs reduce the volume of circulating blood and consequently lower blood pressure. There are more than two dozen different diuretic drugs available and they continue to be widely used as a cheap and moderately effective first line of attack on the problem.

The first modern breakthrough in the field came from one of the greatest drug discoverers of the 20th century, James (later Sir James) Black, in the 1960s. At that time he was working for the pharmaceutical company ICI and he discovered the first of the 'beta-blockers'. These drugs target and block the beta-receptors that are present in the heart. These receptors respond to epinephrine secreted into the blood in conditions of stress from the adrenal gland, and to norepinephrine, a chemical messenger secreted by the nerve fibres that innervate and control the heart.

In either case, stimulation of the beta-receptor causes the heart to increase its rate of contraction and also the strength of each beat. This consequently tends to raise blood pressure. The beta-blockers counteract these effects by preventing the actions of epinephrine and norepinephrine, and consequently they lower blood pressure. In addition, by reducing the amount of work the heart has to do, they are also beneficial in patients suffering from heart failure, a gradual loss of heart function that is common in the elderly. The beta-blockers are often used as a first line of treatment for high blood pressure and heart disease, although they have been superseded by other newer medicines.

Another important advance was the discovery of 'calcium channel blockers'. These drugs act on the muscle that lines the arteries and controls the extent to which the arteries are constricted or relaxed. Obviously it is harder to pump blood through arteries that are constricted, so contraction of the muscle tends to raise blood pressure. An inward movement of the inorganic salt calcium into the cell triggers the contraction of the muscle cells lining the blood vessels, and these drugs act by partially blocking these channels. Consequently they tend to cause the arteries to relax and offer less resistance to blood flow—thus lowering blood pressure. There are many different drugs in this class and they have proved very successful.

A completely different mechanism underlies the therapeutic effects of yet another class of drugs for treating high blood pressure and heart failure, the 'ACE inhibitors'. The hormone angiotensin is one of the most powerful triggers for the contraction of the artery muscles (see Figure 5). It plays a key role in regulating blood pressure and fluid balance in the body. In addition to stimulating the arteries to constrict, angiotensin also acts on the kidneys to suppress urine production, and acts on the brain to stimulate thirst and drinking behaviour. Angiotensin is generated in the blood from an inactive precursor called renin.

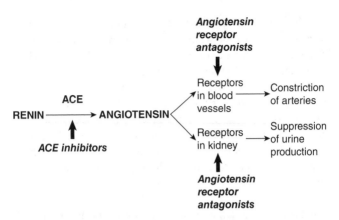

5. How drugs affect biological processes. Drugs that block the synthesis or actions of angiotensin have proved very valuable in treating high blood pressure and heart disease.

The conversion requires an enzyme known as Angiotensin Converting Enzyme (ACE). The idea of using ACE inhibitors to lower blood pressure arose from a discovery in the 1960s by the Brazilian scientist Sergio Ferreira. He observed that the venom of the Brazilian viper caused a profound drop in blood pressure in animals, and tracked this down to a compound in the venom that inhibited this enzyme. Pharmaceutical companies used these discoveries to develop synthetic drugs that act in the same way. The ACE inhibitors proved remarkably effective and safe to use, and, like the beta-blockers, they are used both to lower blood pressure and to protect the failing heart. By the end of the 20th century there were more than a dozen different drugs in this class. Another way of blocking the effects of angiotensin has been to develop drugs that target the receptors in the blood vessels and kidneys on which the hormone acts, rather than preventing its production. A number of angiotensin receptor antagonists have been introduced in recent years, and have proved as effective as the ACE inhibitors—and in some patients they are preferable because of a lower incidence of side effects.

The last category of agents in this area is the cholesterol-lowering drugs. In the Western world, our fat-rich diet and lack of exercise tend to lead to abnormally high blood levels of the fatty substance cholesterol, which accumulates in deposits on the lining of blood vessels, partially blocking them. This in turn increases the risk of high blood pressure, heart failure, and stroke. Less than half of the cholesterol in the blood originates from the diet; the rest is synthesized in the body, mainly in the liver. The cholesterol-lowering drugs, the so-called statins, block this synthesis by targeting a key enzyme in the synthetic pathway: HMG-CoA reductase. In this way it is possible by drug treatment to lower blood cholesterol by as much as 40–50 per cent. The statins were introduced only in the 1980s, but their widespread use became accepted only gradually over the years. They represent a new sort of medicine—one that is taken to prevent a disease from developing, rather than to treat existing symptoms. They do not lower blood pressure or treat the failing heart—but they prevent further cholesterol deposition in the arteries and may even lead to a regression of the deposits that already exist. There is now clear evidence that the statins save lives, particularly in those who have extremely high cholesterol levels or in patients who have already experienced one heart attack. They are among the first widely used 'preventive medicines'. To the pharmaceutical companies, the statins represented a bonanza—once a patient starts taking a statin, he or she will go on doing so for the rest of his or her life. In Western societies perhaps as many as half of all adults have cholesterol levels that might be considered too high. No wonder that the sales of statins when first introduced represented one of the most lucrative classes of prescription medicines, with annual worldwide sales of $13.4 billion in 1999. Today, however, the patents on the original generation of statins have expired, and the cost of these drugs has plummeted. A generic version of simvastatin, one of the original statins, now costs the UK NHS around £1 for a month's supply. The huge reduction in cost has lead to the recommendation from the National Institute of Clinical Excellence (NICE) in the UK (February 2014) that millions more should receive statins, which could prevent thousands of unnecessary deaths from heart attacks or stroke. As far as the NHS is concerned, prevention is far less costly than cure.

The drug treatment of high blood pressure and heart disease is one of the biggest and most successful sectors of the pharmaceutical arena. Many innovative new classes of agents were introduced during the latter half of the 20th century and individual patients can be treated with the most appropriate cocktail of drugs for their particular condition.

Healing gastric ulcers

The stomach is a remarkable organ. When food enters the stomach, the cells lining the stomach secrete a digestive fluid that contains quite a high concentration of hydrochloric acid and is consequently highly acidic. The gastric fluid also contains digestive enzymes, such as pepsin, that can function in this unusually acidic environment. The acidic gastric fluid helps to start the rapid chemical breakdown of foodstuffs, and at the same time sterilizes the food by destroying most of the potentially harmful microorganisms that it may contain. But using such a strong acid secretion carries its own hazards. The cells lining the stomach are protected against acid-induced damage by a thick layer of mucus. However, under some conditions this defence may be broken down, and the resulting exposure of the tender lining of the organ to the acid contents can lead to irritation and eventually to ulcers—painful areas of damaged tissue. Ulcers are particularly likely to occur if too much acid is secreted in the stomach—particularly when food is not present. Such conditions can occur in response to stress of various kinds—and modern life in big cities is full of stress. Excessive intake of alcohol can also damage the protective lining of the stomach, and such intake of alcohol is also a widespread feature of our society. Another risk factor for some people is the irritant effect of aspirin and aspirin-like drugs on the stomach lining. Not surprisingly, stomach ulcers are common.

Prior to the discovery of effective anti-ulcer drugs, the only treatment for severe stomach ulcers was the surgical removal of the damaged part of the stomach. The introduction of powerful new classes of anti-ulcer drugs during the 1970s and 1980s, however, has effectively put the gastric surgeons out of business.

The first breakthrough came again from Sir James Black in the 1970s. It had been known for some time that in the stomach the chemical messenger molecule histamine plays a key role in the train of events leading to gastric acid secretion. The intake of food triggers a release of histamine, which activates the acid-secreting cells. The classical anti-histamine drugs fail to block the actions of histamine in the stomach. James Black showed that this was because histamine acted on a different type of receptor in the stomach from those in skin or lung. He and his colleagues went on to develop the first effective antagonist drugs acting on the so-called histamine H2 receptors in the stomach, and showed that these compounds were very effective in suppressing gastric acid secretion. This in turn helped to heal stomach ulcers, and the H2 blockers became a very successful new class of prescription drugs. James Black won the Nobel Prize in Physiology or Medicine in 1988 for this and his earlier work on beta-blockers. The huge sales of one drug in particular, ranitidine (sold under the trade name Zantac®), helped to lift the British pharmaceutical company Glaxo into the world league. The patent lives of the first H2 blockers have expired, but they continue to enjoy large sales as 'over-the-counter' medicines.

A second breakthrough soon followed in this field with the advent of a new class of drugs that act directly on the acid-secreting cells in the stomach to inhibit acid formation—the so-called 'proton-pump inhibitors'. These drugs are even more effective than the H2 blockers in almost completely suppressing gastric acid secretion. They consequently can help to heal gastric ulcers even more rapidly—with complete healing commonly seen after only one month of drug treatment. The first successful drug of this class was omeprazole (sold under the trade name Losec®), and it helped to change the medium-sized Swedish pharmaceutical company Astra, which discovered it, into a major player in the pharmaceutical industry. The combined annual worldwide sales of the H2 blockers and proton pump inhibitors of nearly $16 billion in 1999 made this one of the most commercially important of all the categories of prescription drugs at that time. However, now that the original patents on these drugs have expired generic versions are available at greatly reduced prices. The current costs of omeprazole or ranitidine to the NHS are £1–2 per month.

These are not the only medicines that are important in the treatment of gastric ulcers. One puzzling feature of the successful treatment of ulcers with H2 blockers or proton-pump inhibitors is that after some time, when the ulcers have healed and the drug treatment stopped, some patients suffer a recurrence. Is this simply because the drugs do not remove the stress that is the underlying cause, or are there other factors? The answer came as a big surprise, in the form of a newly discovered bacterium *Helicobacter pylori*, an organism that has evolved to adapt to the harsh conditions inside the stomach. Two doctors in Australia, Barry Marshall and Robin Warren, who were the first to isolate and identify the bacterium, made the discovery. It had long been assumed that the highly acidic environment of the stomach could not support any life form. But *H. pylori* lives in the protective mucous lining of the stomach, and it has evolved a special enzyme that allows it to generate ammonia as a means of neutralizing the stomach acid. It took more than a decade for the existence of *H. pylori* as a precipitating factor in stomach ulcers to be acknowledged. But it is now clear that the bacterium, by secreting toxic materials, helps to trigger damage to the stomach in many of the patients who develop ulcers. The bacterium is also common, however, in people who do not develop stomach ulcers—almost half of 40-year-old adults in Britain or the USA carry it. It appears to be the presence of *H. pylori*, along with other factors, such as stress or alcohol that does the damage. Nowadays, gastric ulcers are routinely treated with H2 blockers or proton-pump inhibitors, along with an antibiotic to eradicate the *H. pylori* infection. Treatment with bismuth salts, or other drugs that help strengthen the mucous protective coating of the stomach, may also be given as part of a 'triple cocktail'.

Cancer treatment

Cancer remains a common and dreaded disease. Cancer represents an uncontrolled division and growth of tissue cells, resulting in solid tumours or circulating cancer cells which overwhelm the body's defences. It comes in many varieties (see Table 1), often associated with one of the body organs, thus 'lung cancer' is one of the commonest—reflecting in large part the consequence of the popularity of cigarette smoking earlier in the 20th century.

Established approaches to treatment

Among well-established approaches that are still widely used are: surgery—to remove all or part of a cancer; radiotherapy—using high energy rays focused on a cancer to destroy it; and chemotherapy—involving the administration of toxic drugs to kill or inactivate rapidly dividing cells. A wide range of such chemicals is approved for this use, and they may prove very effective. There are serious adverse side effects, however, including severe nausea and vomiting that are common during the treatment and for several days thereafter. Since the drugs target rapidly dividing cells they will also adversely affect body tissues which contain such cells—these include the hair follicles, bone marrow, skin, and the lining of the gut. Thus chemotherapy commonly leads to a loss of hair and damage to the immune system that is normally reliant on bone marrow for its cells. Surgical transplants of stem cells and bone marrow may accompany chemotherapy to reduce such risks.

Table 1 Prevalence and deaths annually in USA associated with the commonest forms of cancer

Cancer type	Estimated new cases	Estimated deaths
Bladder	74,000	16,000
Breast	231,840	40,290
Colon and rectal (combined)	132,700	49,700
Endometrial	54,870	10,170
Kidney cancer	61,560	14,080
Leukaemia (all types)	54,270	24,450
Lung (including bronchus)	221,200	158,040
Melanoma	73,870	9,940
Non-Hodgkin lymphoma	71,850	19,790
Pancreatic	48,960	40,560

Source: Data from US National Cancer Institute January 2015

Targeted cancer therapies

Targeted cancer therapies are drugs or antibodies that block the growth and spread of cancer by interfering with specific molecules that are involved in the growth, progression. and spread of cancer. These are sometimes called 'molecularly targeted therapies'.

The development of targeted cancer therapies requires the identification of molecules that play a key role in cancer cell growth and survival. Proteins that are present in cancer cells but not in normal cells, or which are present in unusually large amounts, might be targets, especially if they are known to be involved in cell growth or survival. For example, 'human epidermal growth factor receptor 2 protein' (HER-2) is expressed at high levels on the surface of some cancer cells. Several targeted therapies are directed against HER-2, including one of the first monoclonal antibodies trastuzumab ('Herceptin®'). Another approach is to identify mutant (altered) proteins that drive cancer progression. For example, the cell growth signalling protein BRAF is present in an altered form (known as BRAF-V600E) in many melanomas, and the monoclonal antibody vemurafenib ('Zelboraf®') is effective in treating melanomas that contain this mutant protein. Not all targeted cancer therapies are monoclonal antibodies, for example imatinib ('Gleevec®') is a synthetic chemical that targets the BCR-ABL fusion protein which promotes growth of some leukemia cells.

The development of targeted cancer therapies is now a sophisticated technical process, involving the automated screening of numerous drug molecules or antibodies against a potential target (see Table 2).

Targeted therapies are a big step forward, but they are not always effective. Cancer cells often become resistant to treatment, either because the target itself mutates, or the cancer cells use a new pathway to achieve tumour growth. For this reason, targeted treatment often combines two targeted medicines, or a targeted medicine with a conventional treatment such as chemotherapy.

The treatment of cancer has improved greatly in the past 40 years, partly because of better early diagnosis, but also because of the wide variety of targeted treatments now available. Half of the patients diagnosed with any cancer in the period 2010–11 in England and Wales will survive for ten years. This overall figure includes wide ranges in ten-year survival rates, from 98 per cent for testicular cancer, to only 5 per cent for lung cancer. Overall in England and Wales survival rates have doubled in the past forty years. Survival rates in some European countries, and in the USA, have improved even more. The increased availability of

Table 2 Approved medicines for some cancer targets

Cancer	Approved medicines
Breast	Everolimus (Affinitor®); tamoxifen (Fareston®); trastuzimab (Herceptin®); fulvestrant (Faslodex®); anastrozole (Arimidex®); exemestane (Aromosin®); lapatinib (Tykerb®); letrozole (Femara®); pertuzumab (Perjeta®); adotrastuzumab emtansine (Kadcyla™); palbociclib (Ibrance®)
Colo-rectal	Cetuximab (Erbitux®); panitumumab (Vectibix®); bevacizumab (Avastin®); ziv-aflibercept (Zaltrap®); regorafenib (Stivarga®)
Kidney	Bevacizumab (Avastin®); sorafenib (Nexavar®); sunitinib (Sutent®); pazopanib (Vortrient®); everolimus (Afinitor®); axtinib (Inlyta®)
Leukaemia	Tretinoin (Vesanoid®); imatinib mesylate (Gleevac®); dasatinib (Sprycel®); nilotinib (Tasigna®); bosutinib (Bosulif®); rituximab (Rituxan®); alemtuzumab (Campath®); ofatumumab (Arzerra®); obinutuzumab (Gazyva®); ibrutinib (Imbruvica®); idelalisib (Zydelig®); binatumomab (Blincyto®)
Lung	Bevacizumab (Avastin®); crizotinib (Xalcori®); erlotinib (Tarceva®); gefitinib (Iressa®); afatinib dimaleate (Gilotrif®); ceritinib (Zycadia); ramucirumab (Cyramaza®); nivolumab (Opdivo®)
Lymphoma	Ibritumomab tiuxetan (Zevalin®); denileukin difitox (Ontak®); brentuximab vedotin (Adcetris®); rituximab (Rituxan®); vorinostat (Zolinza®); romidepsin (Istodax®); bexarotene (Targretin®); bortezomib (Velcade®); pralatrexate (Folotyn®); lanaliomide (Revlimib®); ibrutinib (Imbruvica®); siltuximab (Sylvant™); idelalsib (Zdelig®); belinostat (Beleodaq®)
Melanoma	Ipilimumab (Yervoy®); vemurafenib (Zelboraf®); trametinib (Meklinist®); dabrafenib (Tafinlar®); pembrolizumab (Keytruda®); nivolumab (Opdivo®);
Pancreas	Erlotinib (Tarceva®); everolimuis (Afinitor®); sunitinib (Sutent®)

Source: Selected data from US National Cancer Institute <http://www.cancer.gov/cancertopics/treatment/types/target-therapie> 'What targeted therapies have been approved for specific types of cancer' (reviewed April 2014).

Note: those names ending in '—inib' are inhibitors of one or other of the large family of protein kinase enzymes; those ending in '—mab' are monoclonal antibodies.

monoclonal antibodies to treat specific cancers is likely to have a further beneficial effect on treatment outcome in the future.

Combating pain and inflammation

The immune system represents an immensely complex system of defence mechanisms that are called into play to counteract infections or injuries. The immune system is programmed to recognize any foreign materials and to activate the various defence mechanisms that are designed to destroy invading microorganisms or to repair tissue damage. It does so by mobilizing antibodies—proteins that recognize foreign proteins or other large molecules—and helping to inactivate them. Binding of the foreign materials to antibodies helps to accelerate their disposal by the various classes of white blood cells, which attack, kill, and eventually engulf foreign cells or invading microorganisms. White cells leave the bloodstream and concentrate in regions of tissue injury, where they help to remove dead and damaged cells and set up a local inflammatory response that is often painful. The immune system and white cells communicate with each other and with the rest of the body by means of a complex family of chemical signalling molecules known as chemokines and cytokines. These include a large family of proteins known as the interleukins and others with such exotic names as 'tumour necrosis factor' and 'interferons'. These molecules are generated when the immune system is activated and, among other things, they act on the brain to cause the so-called sickness syndrome, characterized by fever, sleepiness, and loss of appetite, symptoms that are well known to anyone who has suffered from a bout of flu or other infectious disease. Until recently it was not possible to interfere with the complex molecular machinery underlying inflammation, but monoclonal antibodies have been developed which do just that, and these have proved to be a major advance, as discussed later in this section.

The immune system plays an essential role in combating enemies that would otherwise destroy us, but this powerful defence system can also go wrong and turn against itself. A number of common human illnesses represent 'autoimmune' disorders, in which for some reason the immune system no longer recognizes some part of the body as 'self' and initiates an attack, with consequent inflammation and damage. Examples include arthritis, where joints become inflamed and painful and the cartilage and bone are gradually eroded; multiple sclerosis, a progressive disease of the nervous system in which the fatty material called myelin, which wraps around and insulates nerve fibres, is gradually attacked; and asthma, in which a chronic inflammation is set up in the lungs, leading to difficulties in breathing.

Fortunately there are many drugs available to treat the symptoms of pain and inflammation. One of the oldest and most widely used of all drugs is aspirin. Aspirin is the drug name given to the chemical substance acetylsalicylic acid. It is a good example of how a relatively minor change in the parent chemical, salicylic acid, can lead to a dramatic improvement. The beneficial effects of extracts of willow bark (*Salix alba*) in reducing fevers were known since the 18th century, and by the 1870s the effects of willow bark had been traced to the chemical salicylic acid. Methods for synthesizing salicylic acid were developed in Germany, and the Heyden Chemical Company initiated the commercial marketing of it as a medicine. It became widely used not only for fevers, but also for its effectiveness in reducing the pain associated with rheumatism, arthritis, headaches, and neuralgias. Salicylic acid, however, was far from the ideal medicine—it was administered as a solution with a vile and bitter taste, which often caused the patient to vomit, and it caused severe irritation to the lining of the stomach that could lead to life-threatening bleeding ulcers. It was the chemist Felix Hoffmann and the pharmacologist Heinrich Dreser, working in the Bayer Company in Germany, who solved these problems in 1898 by synthesizing the acetyl derivative of salicylic acid, aspirin. In a scientific paper published in 1899 Dreser showed that in animals aspirin retained the excellent pain-relieving and fever-reducing properties of the parent substance and at the same time offered a safer and more convenient medicine, patented by the Bayer Company in 1899. Aspirin lacks the bitter taste of the parent salicylic acid, but does not dissolve readily in water, and so the Bayer Company decided to supply the compound in the form of compressed tablets, which would disintegrate into powder form in the stomach. Aspirin thus became the first major medicine to be sold in tablet form. Launched at the turn of the 20th century, it became the 'drug of the century'. Aspirin was widely used to treat many sorts of pain, and the availability of a safe and non-addictive painkiller was very welcome at a time when morphine was the only alternative available. For a while the Bayer Company enjoyed a monopoly position and reaped huge commercial profits from the drug, although Germany forfeited many of the aspirin-related patents at the end of World War I. After 1918 many other companies were able to manufacture and market the drug, as the original patents were forfeited. This led to intensely competitive marketing campaigns, the so-called 'aspirin wars', to sell what became one of the most widely used of all medicines (see Figure 6).

New medical uses continue to be discovered for aspirin. One of its many effects is to act on specialized cells in the blood known as platelets, which are important in blood clotting. By disabling the platelet-clotting mechanism, aspirin makes blood less likely to clot—and, since unwanted blood clots can initiate heart attacks or a stroke, taking a low dose of aspirin every day is recommended to patients who are at risk of these events. The mechanism underlying the actions of aspirin remained unknown until the British pharmacologist John (later Sir John) Vane and his colleagues showed in 1971 that it acts as an inhibitor of a key enzyme in the inflammatory mechanism called cyclooxygenase. This enzyme generates an inflammatory mediator known as prostaglandin, which triggers pain and other aspects of inflammation. By inhibiting the formation of prostaglandin, aspirin reduces pain and dampens down the overall inflammatory process. Vane showed that not only aspirin but all the other

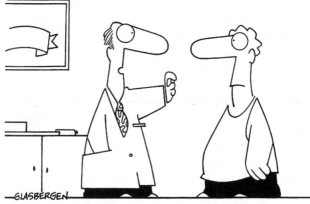

"To prevent a heart attack, take one aspirin every day.
Take it out for a jog, then take it to the gym,
then take it for a bike ride...."

6. Aspirin cartoon.

so-called non-steroidal anti-inflammatory drugs (NSAIDs) that had been developed since aspirin (for example, ibuprofen, etoflac, and indomethacin) also worked by the same mechanism. Vane was awarded the Nobel Prize in Physiology or Medicine in 1982 in recognition of this seminal discovery.

The aspirin story continued to develop. A new class of NSAIDs was introduced at the end of the 20th century that were as effective as the previous drugs as pain-relievers and anti-inflammatory agents, but were much less prone to cause gastric irritation and bleeding, which remain the most common and serious of the unwanted side effects associated with aspirin and the other aspirin-like drugs. Although these side effects are rarely serious, they can become so, and, because so many millions of people take aspirin and other NSAIDS, several thousand people die each year as a result of severe drug-induced gastric bleeding. The new drugs target a newly discovered form of the cyclooxygenase enzyme, known as COX-2. Unlike the previously studied enzyme, now known as COX-1, the COX-2 enzyme is generated only in response to inflammation or injury. It is thus an ideal target for anti-inflammatory drugs. Unlike the older NSAIDS, which inhibit both enzymes equally, the new drugs selectively inhibit only the COX-2 enzyme. The COX-2 enzyme is not present in the cells lining the stomach where COX-1 is found, so the COX-2 inhibitors do not cause gastric irritation and bleeding. The COX-2 inhibitors looked set to be as successful in the 21st century as aspirin had been one hundred years earlier. Sales of the two COX-2 blockers launched at the turn of the century refecoxib ('Vioxx®') and celecoxib ('Celebrex®'), already exceeded $3 billion in 2000 and another COX-2 antagonist valdecoxib ('Bextra'), was launched. However, the celebrations were short-lived. Long-term clinical trials revealed that patients treated with 'Vioxx' suffered a significantly increased risk of heart attacks or stroke—in light of which 'Vioxx' was withdrawn from the market. 'Bextra' was similarly withdrawn and the US Food and Drug Administration imposed detailed warnings to be given to all patients receiving 'Celebrex', or older NSAIDs—which also carried some similar risk.

Other aspirin-like drugs exist, the most widely used of which is acetaminophen ('paracetamol' in Europe, marketed as 'Panadol' or 'Tylenol' in USA). Paracetamol is an effective painkiller and reduces fevers, but is safer than aspirin. It does not cause gastric irritation and can be given to children or elderly patients. The mechanism of action is somewhat obscure, but it may act by inhibiting the cyclooxygenase enzyme in the brain rather than in peripheral tissues. There is a danger, however, as in an overdose paracetamol can cause serious damage to the liver and kidneys. Because it is so widely used, there are paracetamol-related deaths every year—sometimes as a result of deliberate suicidal overdosing.

The real blockbusters for the 21st century, however, are monoclonal antibodies that target a key protein in the inflammatory cascade, the cytokine 'tumour necrosis factor-α' (TNF-α). By binding to TNF-α the antibodies disrupt its function, and inhibit the overall process of inflammation. They are given by injection—often supplied in a 'pen' that patients can use to inject themselves subcutaneously. Because the antibodies persist for some time in the circulation they need be given only at weekly or biweekly intervals. The clinical results for some patients suffering from inflammatory diseases such as rheumatoid arthritis have often been spectacular. Chronic pain and swelling that the patient has suffered for many years can suddenly be reversed. Several products of this type are currently available: infliximab ('Remicade'), etanercept ('Enbrel'), adalimumab ('Humira') and golimumab ('Simponi'). These products have radically changed the treatment of inflammatory illnesses, but they come at a price—literally. The major drugs listed here cost \$20–25,000 per patient per annum in the USA. In Europe national health schemes have struggled to meet such costs. In Britain the National Health Service (NHS) pays £9,300 (\$13,500) per annum for the leading product 'Humira', and it is only prescribed for serious cases where other medicines have failed. These new drugs have become hugely successful both clinically and commercially; in 2014 'Humira' was no. 2 in the USA Sales Chart, earning \$6 billion, and 'Enbrel' was no. 4, earning \$4.3 billion. High prices have been characteristic of the market for monoclonal antibodies, which have made dramatic impacts in other branches of medicine. There is some prospect that this will prove only a temporary phenomenon, however. The European Medicines Agency (EMA), which is responsible for approving all new medicines, has defined the rules for approving 'biosimilar' products. Although no two antibodies can ever be exactly the same in their molecular structure, an antibody that targets the same protein as the original monoclonal antibody, and does so in a similar, if not identical, way at the molecular level, and is as effective clinically can be approved as a form of 'generic' when the original patents on monoclonal antibodies expire. This is beginning to happen: the EMA have approved the first 'biosimilars' 'Inflectra' and 'Remsima' to compete with off-patent

'Remicade'. Although these have not yet been approved in the USA, they are marketed at a saving of around 30 per cent in Europe.

For more severe forms of pain, often associated with such terminal illnesses as cancer, morphine, or morphine-like drugs, the 'opiates', remain the most effective options. (Opiates are analgesics derived from the opium poppy (natural); opioids are analgesics that are at least part synthetic, not found in nature). Morphine acts on specific opiate receptor sites in the brain and spinal cord to dampen the flow of nerve impulses in nerve tracts that carry 'pain' information into the brain. These receptors are not there to recognize the plant-derived drug, but they are part of the body's own pain defence system. The opiate receptors are normally activated by naturally occurring chemicals known as endorphins (*end*ogenous m*orphines*). These chemicals are released particularly in conditions of stress or emergency when 'fight or flight' is more important than feeling pain. Thus, the footballer injured on the field or the soldier wounded in battle does not feel the pain immediately. There are now many synthetic chemical drugs that act on the same receptors as morphine, and some of these are many times more potent than morphine itself (for example, fentanyl). Morphine itself, however, continues to be widely used, and new slow-release preparations (e.g. fentanyl skin patch) make it possible to control most forms of pain with a drug regime that administers a dose at most once or twice a day. There are problems associated with the repeated use of morphine and related opiates, however. Doctors are often frightened of using these drugs except in the terminally ill in case they create drug addiction (see Chapter 4). Experience with the morphine-like drug oxycodone ('Oxycontin') shows that this concern is well founded. Since oxycodone was marketed in the USA there has been an epidemic of addicted users. This has not been seen, so far, in Europe—perhaps because obtaining prescription medicines is easier in the USA than in Europe. Another problem with the repeated use of morphine-like drugs is the development of tolerance, so that higher and higher drug doses are needed, and eventually the patient may no longer obtain adequate pain relief. There remains a real need for better medicines to control severe chronic pain.

Treatment of neuropathic pain

Neuropathic pain is distinct from inflammatory pain, and does not respond to NSAIDs or opiates. It occurs when sensory nerves are damaged—which may occur as a result of diabetes, treatment with toxic chemotherapy agents in cancer, or infection with herpes zoster ('shingles'). The sensation is a burning pain, and can be hard to treat. The tricylic antidepressant drugs amitriptyline and imipramine sometimes help pain relief, although not acting not in the way in which they treat depression by boosting monoamine function (see the next section, 'Healing the damaged mind'), but probably by blocking voltage sensitive ion channels on sensory nerves. Other drugs include gabapentin ('Neurontin') and pregabalin ('Lyrica'), despite their names their mechanisms of action do not involve any direct interaction with the inhibitory neurotransmitter GABA, instead they target a particular sub-unit of voltage-sensitive calcium channels in sensory nerves. A particular form of neuropathic pain, in which nerve fibre tracts in the brain are damaged, affects some patients with multiple sclerosis (MS). This form of 'central' pain is particularly hard to treat. Recently a standardized extract of cannabis, 'Sativex', has been approved for the treatment of MS pain, the first medical use of cannabis since the 19th century. Neuropathic pain remains a chronic burden for many sufferers; the available drugs provide pain relief for only around half of them.

Healing the damaged mind

One of the most remarkable advances in pharmacology in the latter half of the 20th century was the discovery and widespread use of drugs that help to treat the symptoms of mental disorders.

The availability of drugs that ameliorate the symptoms of schizophrenia, depression, and anxiety has had a major impact on the way in which we view these diseases: they are seen increasingly as having an organic basis. The drugs have also led to radical changes in the management of mental illnesses. They helped to accelerate the closure of mental hospitals as places where dangerous mad people had to be kept locked away from the rest of society.

Virtually all of the drugs used in psychiatry act in one way or another on the chemical messenger systems in the brain (see Figure 7). The billions of nerve cells in the brain communicate with each other in complex neural circuits. Nerve cells maintain a small electrical potential between the inside of the cell and the

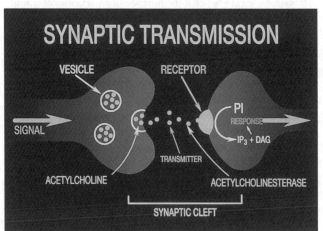

7. **Chemical transmission in the nervous system. Nerve cells (neurons) transmit minute electrical impulses down their cable-like fibres (axons). When the impulses reach the ending of the fibre they trigger the release of bursts of a neurotransmitter chemical which activate the target cell. Many drugs that act on the nervous system do so by either mimicking neurotransmitter molecules or by blocking their actions on target.**

outside world, and the discharge of this 'battery' allows them to transmit electrical impulses along their elongated fibres. When the electrical pulse reaches the vicinity of the next cell in the circuit, however, transmission from cell to cell is no longer electrical but chemical. The nerve impulse arriving at the ending of a nerve fibre causes the discharge of a minute amount of one or other of the many different chemical messenger substances used in the brain. The chemical acts on receptor proteins on the surface of the target cell to cause either an excitation or an inhibition of the activity of that cell (it is as important to have OFF signals as it is to have ON signals).

More than fifty different chemicals are used in this way as messenger molecules, and each is recognized by its own specific cell surface receptors. This offers many different targets for drug intervention, either to boost the function of a particular chemical messenger or to block its actions. The first effective drugs used to treat clinical depression were compounds that act by enhancing the activity of chemicals known as monoamines in the brain. The two chemicals that appear particularly relevant for depression are norepinephrine (noradrenaline) and serotonin. Each of these plays a role in modulating the activity of the thinking part of the brain, the cerebral cortex. Norepinephrine helps to alert the brain to interesting events going on in the outside world, and serotonin plays a key role in determining the emotional state and mood.

The first safe and effective antidepressant drugs were discovered in the 1950s: imipramine in Europe by the Swiss company CIBA-GEIGY, and amitriptyline by the American company Merck. These drugs boost monoamine function in the brain. After release from nerve endings, norepinephrine and serotonin are inactivated by a recapture mechanism whereby they are pumped back into the nerve endings from which they had been released by means of a specific transporter protein located in the cell membrane of the nerve. The antidepressants imipramine and amitriptyline act by inhibiting these amine pump mechanisms, thus prolonging the actions of released monoamines. Dr Julius Axelrod, working at the US National Institute of Mental Health, was the first to discover the monoamine reuptake mechanisms, and the actions of the antidepressants on them—for which he was awarded the Nobel Prize in Physiology or Medicine in 1970. Imipramine and amitriptyline proved hugely popular and continue to be widely used. During the 1980s and 1990s, however, even more successful antidepressants were discovered. These target more selectively just the monoamine transporter for serotonin, leaving other monoamine transporters untouched. The serotonin-selective reuptake inhibitors (SSRIs), epitomized by Prozac® (fluoxetine), are even safer to use than the older drugs, which could prove dangerous in an overdose. Prozac and related SSRIs captured an ever-increasing market for antidepressant medicines—valued at more than $11 billion in 1999. Since then the patents have expired on the original SSRIs, and they have largely been replaced by cheaper generic copies. This has coincided with a massive increase in the use of antidepressants on both sides of the Atlantic, with a 400 per cent increase in the USA, and a 500 per cent increase in Europe during the past twenty years. The availability of safe and effective drugs has demonstrated that clinical depression affects far larger numbers of people than was hitherto thought; the widespread use of these medicines has coincided with a decrease in the rates of suicide in most European countries. Antidepressants have become among the most commonly used of all prescription medicines.

Anxiety often accompanies depression, and it occurs in many different forms. At one extreme are patients who suffer from severe anxiety and panic attacks. They may experience several frightening panic attacks every week, often prompted by some particular phobia—fear of open spaces, or entering the supermarket, or social occasions. There are many milder forms of phobia and anxiety—often associated with generalized anxiety and insomnia. The most effective anti-anxiety drugs (tranquillizers) are the benzodiazepines, epitomized by diazepam (Valium®). The benzodiazepines have a remarkable calming effect on anxious people, and they help to restore normal sleep patterns. Valium® was the best-selling drug in the pharmaceutical world for more than a decade in the 1960s and 1970s, and earned a fortune for the parent Swiss company, Hoffmann la Roche. It was followed by many imitators, all sharing the same pharmacological mechanism, which is to enhance the actions of the key inhibitory brain chemical messenger GABA. Benzodiazepines are also widely used to combat insomnia, and for this purpose very short-acting drugs have been designed—so that they do not leave the patient with a sedated 'hangover' effect on waking next morning. Like most psychopharmaceuticals, however, there is a downside to the repeated use of benzodiazepines. Some patients can become addicted to the drugs, so that they find it difficult to stop taking them. If drug treatment is stopped, it can lead to a period of rebound associated with increased anxiety and sleep disturbance. In Britain it is estimated that thousands of elderly patients remain dependent on prescription benzodiazepines, as a consequence of the freedom with which these were prescribed earlier. On the whole, though, the benzodiazepines represent a remarkably safe group of drugs that have benefited many millions of patients.

We all occasionally suffer from bouts of anxiety or depression, so we feel some empathy for the patients who suffer from the extreme forms of these conditions. The madness of schizophrenia is much more difficult for us to understand. Schizophrenia affects about 1 per cent of the population. It typically develops after puberty in early adult life, and is often a lifelong illness. The symptoms are varied and bizarre; no two patients will be quite the same. Key symptoms include: auditory hallucinations—often hearing voices talking about the patient in the third person; irrational delusions; feelings of persecution and paranoia; inability to express appropriate emotions; incoherent thought processes and language; withdrawal from social contacts and immobility. The illness often leaves the sufferer incapable of normal work or other daily activities, and the delusions may lead the patient to irrational and dangerous acts of violence towards others. The discovery of drugs that tackle some of these key symptoms has been a big advance in the treatment of schizophrenia. The first breakthrough was an accidental discovery. In the early 1950s two French physicians, J. Delay and P. Deniker, noted the remarkable calming effects of a new drug, chlorpromazine, which was initially tested as an agent to be given to patients prior to major surgery to relax them. They tested the drug in patients suffering from mania and found it to be remarkably effective, and this led to tests in schizophrenic patients, where again chlorpromazine had remarkable effects in calming agitated patients, without putting them to sleep—it was a tranquillizer, not a crude sedative. Chlorpromazine rapidly came into widespread use on both sides of the Atlantic as a new and effective treatment for schizophrenia. Many other effective anti-schizophrenia agents followed chlorpromazine, including the very potent drug haloperidol, discovered by the gifted drug-discoverer Paul Janssen in Belgium. Some of these drugs were up to a thousand times more potent than chlorpromazine, so that it proved possible to deliver enough drug to last for several weeks in one single dose—usually given by means of an injection of the drug in an oily fluid into a muscle. This 'depot injection' remains in the muscle and slowly releases an active drug. In this way it has proved possible to treat schizophrenia in outpatient clinics, in which the drug is administered once or twice a month. The availability of such treatments has been one of the factors that led to the gradual disappearance of the Victorian mental hospitals, in which patients with schizophrenia were formerly locked away. However, depot injections are irreversible, and may leave the patient with prolonged adverse effects, and although the anti-schizophrenic drugs can control the symptoms of the disease, they do not alter the natural history of the illness.

Discovering how anti-schizophrenic drugs act in the brain has been one of the achievements of the new subject of 'psychopharmacology', and two of the pioneers in this field, Arvid

Carlsson in Sweden and Paul Greengard in the USA, were awarded the Nobel Prize in Physiology or Medicine in 2000. They helped to show that the key target for all of the effective drugs in this class is one of the monoamine chemical messengers called dopamine. The drugs used to treat schizophrenia, known as neuroleptics, act by blocking the actions of dopamine at one of its receptors in the brain.

Dopamine is also associated with another brain disorder, Parkinson's disease, in which the nerve cells that make and release dopamine gradually degenerate, leaving the sufferer unable to initiate movements, and with rigid limbs often accompanied by a tremor. The drug L-DOPA is used in the treatment of Parkinson's disease; L-DOPA enters the brain where it is converted to dopamine to replace the missing brain chemical. It is thus no surprise to learn that that an overdose of L-DOPA can cause psychotic symptoms, or that one of the adverse side effects of anti-schizophrenic drugs is to cause symptoms similar to those seen in Parkinson's disease. This problem has been largely overcome in a new generation of anti-schizophrenic drugs, which remain as effective as the older drugs in combating the psychotic symptoms of the illness, but are less prone to cause unwanted Parkinsonian side effects. The newer drugs, sometimes called 'atypical neuroleptics', combine the blockade of dopamine receptors with another pharmacological action, blocking one of the receptors used by the monoamine serotonin. By this dual blockade the drugs avoid the Parkinsonian side effects. Schizophrenia is a fairly common illness, and drug treatment, although not a cure, has been of great benefit to millions of patients worldwide.

Much remains to be learned about how drugs act on the brain to produce such dramatic effects on such complex conditions as depression, anxiety, or psychosis. In nearly all cases, for example, the beneficial effects of the drugs are seen only after they have been administered for some weeks—whereas the actual pharmacological action (that is, the blockade of serotonin uptake, the antagonism of dopamine receptors, and so on) is immediate. It seems that the immediate action of the drug triggers some longer-term processes that lead to a gradual correction of mental imbalance—by mechanisms still unknown.

The discovery of new drugs to treat depression, anxiety, and schizophrenia was a major development during the latter half of the 20th century, and many of the new drugs commanded high prices. Although cheap generic copies have become available as patents expired, the field has not seen any really new medicines for decades—and sadly the development of drugs to treat psychiatric disorders is no longer a priority for research in most pharmaceutical companies. Great interest remains, however, in discovering new drugs to treat the growing problem of Alzheimer's disease and other forms of senile dementia, although so far there has been little progress in the pharmacological treatment of dementias (see Chapter 6).

Plagues and pestilences

Throughout human history infectious diseases have plagued us. As the human species became more and more numerous and lived in increasingly high densities in towns and cities, we became a fertile breeding ground for the many species of bacteria, fungi, viruses, and parasites that have evolved specifically to take advantage of *Homo sapiens*. In some cases disease has been spread from animals to man, bubonic plague spread from rat fleas to humans, with disastrous consequences. For most of human history we have had no effective medical means of combating the ravages of infectious diseases, and epidemics of such diseases have proved lethal. The spread of bubonic plague (the 'Black Death'), throughout Europe in the Middle Ages, for example, led to the death of as many as half of the population in many countries. Even in the 20th century, the 'Spanish flu' epidemic killed some thirty million people within six months in 1918—twice as many as had died in World War I.

The German chemist Paul Ehrlich developed the first effective anti-bacterial drug. He experimented with the effects of various chemical substances on disease organisms and in 1910, and found that the 606th compound in a series of synthetic chemicals prepared in his laboratory was effective. The compound contained arsenic, and was called arsphenamine. It was one of the first drugs that effectively killed disease microorganisms, and it inaugurated an era which was to revolutionize the treatment and control of infectious diseases, which had hitherto been largely untreatable. Arsphenamine (sold under the trade name 'Salvarsan') was particularly lethal to the micro-organism responsible for syphilis. Until the introduction of penicillin, 'Salvarsan' (or one of its close chemical relatives that were subsequently developed) remained the standard treatment of syphilis and went a long way towards bringing this social and medical scourge under control.

German chemists learned how to make synthetic dye chemicals that bound strongly to fabrics and could not be removed by washing. They used the same principles to make synthetic medicines that targeted diseases like 'magic bullets', in Ehrlich's famous phrase. In 1932 the German bacteriologist Gerhard Domagk discovered that the red dye Prontosil is active against streptococcal infections in mice and humans. Soon afterward French workers showed that its active antibacterial agent is sulphanilamide. In 1936 the English physician Leonard Colebrook and his colleagues provided overwhelming evidence of the efficacy of both Prontosil and sulphanilamide in streptococcal septicaemia (bloodstream infection), thereby ushering in the sulphonamide era. Domagk and others produced new sulphonamides with astonishing rapidity, many of which had greater potency, wider antibacterial range, or lower toxicity. Domagk was awarded the Nobel Prize in Physiology or Medicine for this work in 1939, but because of his persecution by Nazi Germany he was not able to accept the award until 1947. Some of the new sulpha drugs stood the test of time; others, like the original sulphanilamide and its immediate successor, sulphapyridine, were replaced by safer and more effective successors, many of which are still in use. The sulphonamides represented the first big advance in the war against infectious diseases.

Then followed the era of antibiotics—with the often-told story of Alexander Fleming finding in 1928 that a mould had killed bacteria on an experimental bacterial growth plate left by the window of his laboratory in London. It took another ten years for Howard Florey, Norman Heatley, and Ernst Chain in Oxford to identify the antibacterial substance as penicillin, and to treat the first patient in 1941. Fleming, Florey, and Chain shared the Nobel Prize in Physiology or Medicine in 1945 for their discovery of penicillin. Penicillin proved to be of major importance in World War II in treating infected battle wounds, and production was taken over from war-stricken Britain to America, where the drug was made on a large scale for the first time by Merck and other pharmaceutical companies. Penicillin was to be followed by many other powerful antibiotic drugs, which have revolutionized our ability to combat such killer diseases as pneumonia, tuberculosis, and cholera. The antibiotics were followed in turn later in the 20th century by the first effective drugs for treating virus diseases. How do these miracle drugs work?

Antibacterial and anti-fungal drugs

The ideal drug for treating an infectious disease is one that targets some aspect of biology that is unique to the bacterium or fungus, so that the invading organism can be killed without damaging the human host. The most effective anti-microbial drugs do just that. Bacteria are tiny particles of living matter; they are protected from the outside world by a fairly tough cell membrane—without which they are very vulnerable and cannot survive and multiply. Many antibiotics work by disrupting the ability of the bacteria to synthesize and put together the various sugar and protein components that make up the cell wall. This disables the bacteria, as they cannot reproduce, and the immune system can then clear any remaining infection. Penicillin works in this manner and so do the more than twenty different synthetic analogues of penicillin now available. Another important group of antibiotics, the cephalosporins, a class that includes more than twenty-five different drugs, are chemically distinct from the penicillins but act in the same way as cell wall inhibitors, as do vancomycin and bacitracin.

Other classes of antibacterial agents make use of other differences between bacteria and their hosts. The sulphonamides, for example, interfere with the synthesis of folic acid by bacteria. Folic acid is an essential vitamin that acts as a catalyst for various chemical reactions in all living cells, but, whereas we get the vitamin in our diet, the bacterium must synthesize it. Interfering with this process makes it impossible for the bacteria to grow. Although the sulphonamides were discovered a long time ago, there have been many improvements and some sixteen drugs in this class are still available and widely used. Tetracyclines and the related aminoglycoside antibiotics interfere with another vital life process—the synthesis of proteins. They target the protein synthesis machinery of bacteria, which is different from that of mammals so the drugs do no harm to the host. This class of drugs also includes streptomycin, the first effective antibiotic for the treatment of tuberculosis. The macrolide antibiotics also employ this mechanism of action; this class includes erythromycin, one of the most effective drugs for treating pneumonia. Yet other drugs target the synthesis of nucleic acids by bacteria—another essential feature of life; these include the quinolones and rifampicin.

Infections can be caused by various species of fungi as well as by bacteria. These affect particularly those areas of the body with surfaces exposed to the outside world: skin, lungs, throat, vagina, urinary tract, and so on. Drugs that act against fungal infections, like the antibacterial drugs, target features that are unique to the biology of the invading fungi. As with bacteria, fungi synthesize a tough cell wall and a number of anti-fungal agents interfere with the synthesis or function of this. A cholesterol-like molecule ergosterol, a unique component of fungal cell walls, is a prime target. Amphotericin, nystatin, and imidazoles (e.g. clotrimazole, econazole, miconazole, fluconazole, and ketoconazole) act in this way. Other anti-fungal drugs target features of nucleic acid or protein synthesis unique to fungi.

Drugs to treat virus infections

Taking antibiotics will not cure the common cold, nor will they alleviate the symptoms of flu or influence the course of AIDS infections. These and many other infectious diseases are caused not by bacteria but by viruses. Viruses are the smallest and most simplified forms of life.

Viruses have dispensed with much of the biochemical machinery that other organisms need to live and to reproduce; they do not need this machinery, because they live as parasites within the living cells of their host. Most viruses simply consist of a length of nucleic acid—which carries encoded information about how to make more virus particles—wrapped up in a protein coat. Virus particles infect cells by attaching themselves to the surface of the cell and gaining entry. Once inside the host cell, they shed their protein coat and hijack the biochemistry of the host cell, diverting it to the synthesis of new virus nucleic acid and protein molecules, which will eventually be assembled into millions of new virus particles. The host cell is then killed and the new virus particles released for another round of infection.

Designing effective anti-viral drugs is difficult, as the virus has so few unique features. It uses the normal biochemical machinery of the host, so targeting this is likely to cause damage to the host.

The first effective anti-viral drugs were discovered only in the latter part of the 20th century. Some target the enzyme DNA polymerase, which is needed for the replication of the nucleic acid DNA; without this the virus cannot replicate. But this enzyme is present in all cells of the host. The clever trick here was to design drugs that are not themselves active inhibitors of the DNA polymerase enzyme, but which are selectively converted to such inhibitors only in the virus-infected cells of the host—which contain a viral enzyme that converts the drug. This concept of using an inert drug that is converted in the body to an active agent is an example of the so-called 'pro-drug' strategy. This produced the anti-viral agent acyclovir and a dozen or so later derivatives of it, discoveries that earned the American scientists Gertrude Elion and George Hitchings the Nobel Prize in Physiology or Medicine in 1988. Another important anti-viral drug is zidovudine (AZT); this also impairs the replication of viral nucleic acids, fooling the viral enzyme into incorporating AZT into its own nucleic acid, which can then no longer replicate.

The virus responsible for AIDS, the human immunodeficiency virus (HIV), is one of the most spectacular success stories in viral evolution. This virus has adapted to live in the most numerous large animal on earth (*Homo sapiens*) and it selectively attacks the very cells in the immune system of its host—the T-cells—that are normally in the front line in the body's fight against infections. Furthermore, HIV is spread mainly by sexual contact—one of the most popular forms of human behaviour. The virus gradually destroys the ability of the immune system to mount any further attack, and the body succumbs to the virus and to a variety of other infections—which can include viruses that cause cancers. The first modest success in treating HIV infections came from the use of the anti-viral drugs that target viral nucleic acid replication, but the most successful drugs have emerged in recent years with a different mechanism. They target an enzyme that is unique to the HIV virus. When the virus replicates, the information encoded in the viral nucleic acid is read out as a single long protein, which has to be cut into several different functional protein units. This cutting is done by a special viral enzyme known as HIV protease, and a family of protease inhibitors now represent the most effective drugs in the battle against AIDS. A problem in the treatment of this and other viral diseases is that the virus can mutate to a form that is resistant to the drug. This is evolution running at high speed. During a prolonged period of HIV infection, more than a thousand million particles of HIV virus are generated every day and most are killed by the immune system. The opportunities for a small number of mutant virus particles to arise by chance are thus very high, and if some of these mutants have an advantage, for example, in being resistant to ongoing anti-viral drug treatment, they will survive and multiply. To combat this problem of drug resistance, it is now common to use a protease inhibitor as part of a cocktail of drugs, together with one or more of the earlier anti-viral agents (for example, AZT) to make it more difficult for drug resistance to emerge. This strategy has proved spectacularly successful. In the rich countries of the world AIDS no longer ranks among the top ten causes of death. However, until recently people living in the poorer parts of the world could not afford the expensive drugs used in the West ($10–15,000 per year). This changed radically in the 21st century, with the price of AIDS drugs falling dramatically thanks to reduced prices by Western drug companies, and the availability of cheap 'generic' imitations. The goal of universal access to AIDS drugs by all who need them by 2015 is now realistic.

Killing parasites

As with bacteria, fungi, and viruses, a wide range of parasitic animals have found *Homo sapiens* to be an attractive host in which to live. These range from single-celled organisms, known as Protozoa, to larger parasitic creatures (flatworms, roundworms, hookworms, tapeworms, and so on). Infections are commonest in tropical and subtropical regions, where they can have devastating consequences. The protozoan Trypanosomes, for example, infect cattle in West Africa, making large areas of land unsuitable for cattle farming. In humans, other strains of Trypanosomes invade the brain and cause damage that leads to 'sleeping sickness'. In other tropical countries in Africa, Toxocara or Onchocerca parasitic worms infect the eye and lead to 'river blindness'. A powerful new drug, ivermectin, first discovered as a treatment for the parasites that commonly infect horses and farm animals, can combat the latter condition. Ivermectin has been made available to the World Health Organization (WHO) for a campaign to fight river blindness in Africa in a programme including twenty African countries. A single tablet of this wonder drug taken at six-month intervals can protect children and adults against the terrible consequences of infection with this parasite. In general, though, the pharmaceutical armoury available to treat parasitic infection is not particularly strong. These are diseases that affect mainly the poorer parts of the world, and there is little economic motivation for pharmaceutical companies to invest heavily in research on tropical diseases. The most important example of such neglect is the case of malaria, the commonest and most deadly of all parasitic diseases. Malaria is caused by a group of protozoan parasites known as Plasmodium. Infection is passed from person to person through the bite of an Anopheles mosquito and the parasite grows initially in the liver and then in red blood cells, from which it is eventually released, causing a sudden bout of fever and disability. As many as 200 million people are infected with malaria every year and some half a million of them die from the disease. More than 10,000 cases occur every year in Western tourists visiting malaria-infected regions. Fortunately there are some effective drugs to treat malaria. The oldest of these is quinine, first discovered in the bark of the cinchona tree in the 17th century and later isolated and purified in the 19th century in Paris. Quinine and its derivatives chloroquine and mefloquine kill the malarial parasites in red blood cells by a complex mechanism that involves a chemical reaction with the red blood pigment haemoglobin. Artemisinin, a component of a traditional Chinese medicine, is now widely used to treat malaria. A few other drugs are available: pyrimethamine and proguanil inhibit folic acid synthesis in the parasite—a mechanism similar to that of the sulphonamides in bacteria—and primaquine attacks the parasite in its early stage of development in the liver. Unfortunately, however, drug resistance has become an increasing problem in combating malaria, and in some parts of the world the parasite has already evolved resistance to such an extent that few effective drugs remain available. There is an urgent need to discover new drug treatments for this killer disease.

Resistance to antimicrobials

Antimicrobial resistance (AMR) within a wide range of infectious agents is a growing public health threat of broad concern to countries and multiple sectors. Increasingly, governments around the world are beginning to pay attention to a problem so serious that it threatens the achievements of modern medicine. A post-antibiotic era—in which common infections and minor injuries can kill—far from being an apocalyptic fantasy, is instead a very real possibility for the 21st century.

Dr Fukujda, WHO, 2014

One of the biggest problems in the drug treatment of disease lies in the very area in which there has been such spectacular success in the past century—the use of antibiotics and other drugs to treat infectious diseases. The widespread use of these drugs has led inevitably to the evolution of new strains of bacteria, viruses, and parasites that are drug resistant . That such evolution could occur so rapidly may at first sight seem surprising. However, infectious organisms such as bacteria and viruses grow and reproduce very rapidly in the human body; bacterial numbers can double within a few minutes. During the course of an infection that can last weeks or months, thousands of generations of bacteria will be generated, most of which will be killed by antibacterial drugs or by the immune system. But a tiny proportion of mutant cells that are drug resistant will have an enormous advantage over the others, and they are likely to survive and prosper. Because it is so tempting for doctors to prescribe antibiotics to every patient who turns up with some mild infection and fever, there is a great deal of unnecessary prescribing. In hospitals antibiotics are again almost universally used for sick patients and hospitals have proved to be hotbeds for the evolution and breeding of antibiotic-resistant strains of microorganism, such as methicillin-resistant Staphylococcus aureus (MRSA, Figure 8).

To make matters worse, modern farming methods, in which animals are kept at high densities in confined spaces, are dependent on the widespread use of antibiotics to prevent otherwise inevitable infections. In many cases farm animals are treated indiscriminately with antibiotics to protect them against infections and thus to increase their growth rates.

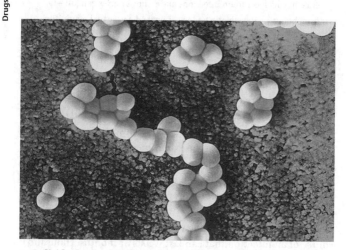

8. Individual cells of the bacterium *Staphylococcus aureus*, greatly enlarged. This bacterium can cause serious infections in wounds or in the lung, leading to pneumonia. Strains of this bacterium that are resistant to many antibiotics are common in modern hospitals.

The molecular devices that microorganisms have evolved to combat antibiotics are truly remarkable. Following the introduction of penicillin, some mutant strains of bacteria started to make a new enzyme 'penicillinase' that was capable of degrading and inactivating the drug. An even more remarkable evolution has been the development of a gene called 'Multiple Drug Resistance' (MDR), which consists of a molecular pump mechanism that can actively expel a number of different antibiotics from the bacterial cell—thus conferring resistance to a whole group of antibiotics. Bacteria have also proved more adept than previously thought in transferring these antibiotic resistant genes from one species of bacteria to another. The evolutionary pressure on the development and spread of these genes has been intense, and so far bacteria have scored ominous successes—making some infectious diseases increasingly difficult to treat. The probability that an in-patient stay in a hospital will lead to an infection with an antibiotic-resistant bacterium is increasing alarmingly every year.

Not only do we face the problem of a post-antibiotic era, but the medicines used to treat fungal, viral, and parasitic diseases are also seeing previously effective medicines rendered ineffective by the development of resistant strains. This is particularly bad news for the treatment of malaria—still a major killer disease in the third world.

Regrettably, pharmaceutical companies have failed to develop any new antibiotics since 1987—partly because it became ever more difficult to discover novel antibiotic mechanisms, and partly because companies saw better commercial opportunities in treating chronic illnesses. Late in the day the prospect of living in a post-antibiotic world, in which infections after a wound or after surgery could prove lethal, has generated an international project coordinated by the WHO to tackle the problem—although who will pay the high costs of developing effective new medicines is not clear.

Few treatments for infectious or parasitic diseases were available until the latter half of the 20th century; by the end of the century several hundred were available. More than any other group of drugs, anti-microbials have affected the health of people who are fortunate enough to live in the developed world; they have largely taken away ancient fears of infectious diseases.

The contraceptive pill

Widely regarded as one of the most important medical advances in the past one hundred years, the 'pill' is now so commonplace that we tend to forget the intense battles that raged over its early days. The 'pill' now exists in more than fifty different products. Most of these contain a progesterone-like synthetic progestin—to suppress the surge in follicle-stimulating hormone (FSH) and luteinizing hormone (LH) that normally triggers ovulation—together with a low dose of a synthetic oestrogen-like substance to suppress breakthrough bleeding. The development of the contraceptive pill relied on three key individuals in 20th-century America. Margaret Sanger was a Catholic whose mother had died at 50, after eighteen pregnancies. This and her experience when training as an obstetrics nurse, working with poor women who had gone through dangerous and harmful abortions, reinforced her view that the contraceptive pill would be important for the safety of women. However, birth control in mid-20th-century society was a taboo subject, which brought Sanger into conflict with the Catholic Church and with 'obscenity laws'. Despite this she founded one of that the first birth control clinics, and formed the Planned Parenthood Federation. Sanger persuaded the endocrinologist Gregory Pincus to carry out research on a contraceptive pill, offering him some support from her charities. Pincus faced an uphill task. Among his more powerful enemies were both the Catholic Church—then, as now, implacably opposed to contraception—and large sections of the political establishment (thanks to Joe McCarthy's war on communism, birth control was widely regarded as part of a Bolshevik conspiracy). Nor was the law on his side. In Massachusetts, where he worked, anyone caught providing contraception faced a possible prison sentence—a situation that persisted until 1972. Research funding for this controversial topic was hard to find, and in 1951 it was the financial support offered by Sanger's friend Katherine McCormick, a wealthy heiress, which proved crucial. The Mexican chemist Karl Djurassi had synthesized progesterone-like substances from Mexican yams and formed the company Syntex. The pharmaceutical company G. D. Searle, although unwilling to support the controversial clinical research, also carried out chemical research on synthetic progestins. Pincus collaborated with Harvard Professor John Rock, and with reproductive physiologist Min Chueh Chang, who was able to test various progestins in animal studies. Pilot clinical studies were aimed initially at treating infertility rather than contraception, but yielded crucial data on the latter. The combination therapy that emerged from this research was the product Enovid, which combined a synthetic progestin norethynodrel with a low dose of the synthetic oestrogen mestranol. Pincus was able to carry out large-scale clinical trials with Enovid in Puerto Rico, where there were no anti-birth control laws. Trials began there in 1956 and were supervised by Dr Edris Rice-Wray. Some of the women experienced side effects from 'the pill', and Rice-Wray wrote to Pincus and reported that Enovid 'gives one hundred percent protection against pregnancy' but causes 'too many side reactions to be acceptable'. Pincus and his colleague Rock disagreed, based on their experience with patients in Massachusetts, and they conducted research showing that placebos caused similar side effects. In May 1960, the FDA approved Enovid, the first contraceptive pill, marketed by G. D. Searle & Co.

This was a momentous event; it presaged the 1960s, the decade of sexual liberation, the sexual revolution, drug culture, rock and roll, and, most importantly, the women's movement. Within a few years of the first FDA approval, millions of women worldwide were taking the pill, and there was an increasing list of contraceptive products available.

There was still concern about adverse side effects. In 1969 Barbara Seaman published 'The Doctor's Case Against the Pill', which reported serious side effects including the risk of blood clots, heart attack, stroke, depression, weight gain, and loss of libido. The controversy over serious side effects, especially thrombosis (blood clots) continued for many years. By 1979 sales of contraceptive pills in the USA had dropped by 24 per cent. This issue was clarified by the data from a series of clinical trials involving thousands of women treated with the 'pill' for many years, which were published in the *British Medical Journal* in August, September and October 2009. The conclusion was that there is a small but significant increase in the risk of thrombosis which affected a small minority of users. The risk of thrombosis in untreated women is around 5 per 100,000, and this was increased by between threefold and fivefold in women taking the pill. The use of oral contraceptives containing levonorgestrel was associated with the lowest incidence of thrombosis. The risk of a serious adverse effect in less than 1 in 1,000 women has to be weighed against the risk of unwanted pregnancy.

For women who want to become pregnant someday, but not immediately, long-acting reversible contraception is available. This offers effective birth control with little day-to-day hassle. Options include a contraceptive implant (e.g. 'Nexplanon', 'Norplant'), or a depot injection of medroxyprogesterone acetate (DMPA) (e.g. 'Depo-Provera'). Some have advocated the use of long-acting reversible contraception for adolescent girls, to help decrease the teenage pregnancy rate, but this raises ethical concerns.

Overall, the success of contraceptive medicines has been remarkable—not many medicines are associated with 100 per cent efficacy! It is not surprising that control over such a fundamental natural process as pregnancy has raised numerous debates and concerns, but the fact that most women in the developed world, and an increasing number in the developing world, practise contraception is a tribute to the early pioneers who made this possible. Indeed it could be argued that contraception has proved too effective in several countries which face declining populations as the replacement rate has fallen below the two children per family required for stability. Without substantial numbers of immigrants entering the USA and Europe, the problem of declining populations would have become more acute.

Chapter 4
Recreational drugs

People in both rich and poor countries seem to have a constant desire to alter their state of consciousness. They use stimulant drugs that allow them to stay awake and dance the night away, sedatives to calm their anxieties, and intoxicants to experience new forms of consciousness and to forget the troubles of everyday life.

The problem is that recreational drug use can lead to abuse. One of the insidious aspects of recreational drug use is that it can all too easily lead to the user becoming addicted to the drug. The symptoms of addiction may include 'tolerance' (the need to take larger and larger doses of the substance to achieve the desired effect), and 'physical dependence' (an altered physical state induced by the substance that produces physical 'withdrawal symptoms', such as nausea, vomiting, seizures, and headache, when substance use is terminated); but neither of these is necessary or sufficient for the diagnosis of addiction. Addiction can be defined in some instances entirely in terms of 'psychological dependence'.

The addicted drug-user may continue to take excessive amounts of the drug, even though it is clearly damaging to work, health, and family. Fortunately, not everyone who takes a recreational drug becomes dependent on it. It is possible that there are people with an 'addictive personality' who are more susceptible than others. Drugs differ in their addiction liability—ranging from high risk in the case of cocaine, heroin, and nicotine to lower risk in the case of alcohol, cannabis, and amphetamines. The process of addiction does not depend entirely on the drug, it requires the repeated use of a drug over prolonged periods, so scientists think of it as involving a change in the pattern of genes that are switched on (or off) in the brain, but just what the critical changes are is not yet clear. Animals can become dependent on recreational drugs, and research on animal brains has suggested that there may be some common mechanisms that are triggered by a number of different drugs. Although the primary sites of action of heroin, amphetamines, nicotine, cocaine, and cannabis in the brain are all different, these drugs share an ability to promote the release of the chemical messenger dopamine in certain brain regions. Although this is not necessarily akin to triggering a 'pleasure' mechanism, it is thought that the drug-induced release of dopamine may be an important signal that prompts the animal or person to seek continued drug use.

Alcohol

Alcohol is the oldest of all recreational drugs, and it is widely consumed in the Western world. The production of wines, beers, and distilled spirits is a very large industry, with worldwide sales in 2015 of more than $1 trillion (approximately the same as the global sales of all medicines). In most Western countries more than 80 per cent of the adult population will admit to having tried alcohol, and about 50 per cent are regular users. The consumption of alcohol continues to increase; in many countries alcoholic products are available twenty-four hours a day in supermarkets. The alcohol industry spends large amounts of money on advertising to encourage the sales of its products. The consumption of alcoholic drinks is deeply embedded in the culture of many countries: the special atmosphere of the traditional English pub or the German beer garden; the custom of drinking wine with the meal in France and Italy; the ice-cold aquavit of the Scandinavian cold table; and the universal champagne at the wedding reception.

Exactly how alcohol acts in the brain to produce initially a state of excitement and intoxication and later sedation is not precisely understood. Scientists believe that the key actions of alcohol target the two principal chemical messenger systems in the neural circuits of the brain. Alcohol enhances the actions of the main OFF signal, GABA, and partially blocks the main ON signal, L-glutamate. But there is more to it than that: the pleasurable intoxicant actions of alcohol seem to be due in part to its ability to stimulate opiate mechanisms in the brain—the same ones that are stimulated more directly and more aggressively by heroin. The drug naltrexone, which acts as an antagonist of the opiate receptors in the brain, has been used successfully in treating heroin addicts, and it has been shown to be effective in treating alcoholics. The drug removes the pleasurable effects of both heroin and alcohol, making it easier for the dependent user to quit.

The majority of drinkers are able to indulge in alcohol without damaging themselves or others, but alcohol consumption also has a considerable downside (see Box 4). The acute stage of alcohol intoxication releases normal inhibitions and tends to promote reckless sexual behaviour, and violent behaviour. Fights with broken bottles and beer glasses as weapons can interrupt the friendly atmosphere of the English pub. In addition, the adverse effects of the drug on the regions of the brain that are involved in behaviours that require precise control, as in driving a motor vehicle, make it dangerous to drink and drive. A very high proportion (more than 50 per cent) of fatal traffic accidents is associated with alcohol. A high proportion of violent crimes, in particular domestic violence, are also associated with drinking.

A certain proportion, perhaps as many as 5–10 per cent, of users become dependent on the drug as alcoholics. Alcohol will come to dominate their lives, often leading to loss of job and family. They may suffer physical damage to the liver (cirrhosis) and other organs, and in extreme cases they may suffer drug-induced brain damage and premature dementia. It is estimated that there are 150,000 alcohol-related deaths in the USA each year.

The consumption of alcohol during pregnancy poses special risks. About 1 in 1,000 of the children born in the USA every year suffer from 'foetal alcohol syndrome'. This is a condition in which the development of the brain is permanently impaired, and it leads to permanent retardation of intellect, with IQ scores of 60 or less. Foetal alcohol syndrome is the single most important cause of mental retardation in the USA.

Nicotine

Nicotine is the drug present in tobacco products or 'electronic cigarettes' that is responsible for their pleasurable qualities. The drug acts in the brain on receptors for the chemical messenger acetylcholine. The nerve tracts that release acetylcholine in the brain have among their functions the ability to act as an alerting or arousal system for the cerebral hemispheres—the thinking part of the brain. Smokers say that it helps them to think more clearly and that nicotine has a mild anti-anxiety property.

Nicotine is not absorbed well when swallowed, but it can be absorbed by chewing, because of the mildly alkaline conditions in the oral cavity, however it is most efficiently delivered by smoking. The burning tobacco converts the nicotine into a vapour that condenses into tiny droplets that are inhaled as a smoke and rapidly absorbed into the blood from the large surface area of the lungs. Smoking delivers nicotine to the brain within seconds of lighting the cigarette. Experienced smokers learn to vary the frequency of puffs and the depth of inhalation to deliver exactly the amount of drug that they want. Unfortunately, smoking also confers special dangers because of the many toxic chemicals present in tobacco smoke. Apart from chemicals already present in the tobacco, new highly toxic cancer-producing chemicals (carcinogens) are created in the process of burning. In addition, cigarette smoke contains an appreciable amount of the gas carbon monoxide (a product of incomplete combustion), which poisons the blood pigment haemoglobin, making it less able to carry oxygen. The latter effect is thought to be one of the principal reasons why mothers who smoke during pregnancy tend to have low birth weight babies—because the foetus is constantly starved of oxygen.

More serious consequences result from the effects of tobacco smoke on the lungs. In the short term these include an increased risk of bronchitis and other forms of obstructive lung disease, and in the longer term an increased risk of cardiovascular disease and lung cancer. The discovery of the link between cigarette smoking and lung cancer was one of the great achievements of medical research of the 20th century. The initial reports in 1950 from Britain and the USA were followed by many other studies. The findings are alarming: not only is the risk of dying from lung cancer increased in cigarette-smokers, but so are the risks of dying from twenty-three other causes, including cancers of the mouth, throat, larynx, pancreas, and bladder and such obstructive lung diseases as asthma and emphysema. It is hard to overestimate the importance of tobacco smoking as the principal avoidable cause of death in the modern world. More people die from smoking tobacco than any other single cause. Worldwide some six million deaths a year can be attributed to tobacco. People in the developing countries started smoking later in the 20th century, but they are catching up fast in the tobacco mortality statistics. Cigarette smoking in China has increased dramatically in the recent past—almost quadrupling since 1980. Cigarette smoking first became common among men in the developed world during the early years of the 20th century, and adverts promoted its health benefits. It was not until thirty or forty years later that the first evidence of a link between tobacco smoking and lung cancer was obtained. Such long lag periods between cause and effect are hard to comprehend. The relationship between cigarette smoking and lung cancer is very complex, and has been well documented by a longitudinal study of more than 50,000 GPs in the UK. The increased risk of developing lung cancer depends far more strongly on the duration of cigarette smoking than on the number of cigarettes consumed each day. Thus, while smoking three times as many cigarettes a day does increase the lung-cancer risk approximately threefold, smoking for thirty years as opposed to smoking for fifteen years does not simply double the lung cancer risk, it increases the risk by twentyfold; and smoking for forty-five years as opposed to fifteen years increases the lung cancer risk one hundredfold (see Figure 9).

The well-documented health risks associated with smoking cigarettes finally triggered a major change in smoking behaviour. New laws in Europe and the USA banned smoking in all public spaces, including bars and restaurants. It may be hard to imagine a ban on smoking in an Irish pub—but this has happened. There has been a sharp drop in the prevalence of cigarette smoking, and an increase in the number of smokers seeking to quit the habit.

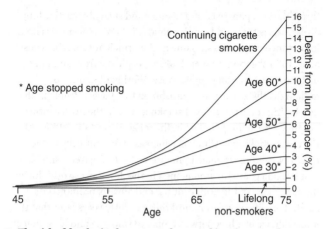

9. The risk of developing lung cancer from smoking cigarettes decreases if smokers quit; the earlier they quit the lower the cancer risk.

There is a clear psychological withdrawal syndrome experienced by smokers who try to quit—it includes agitation, nervousness, bad temper, and a craving for nicotine. The most successful treatment for smokers trying to quit is to satisfy their craving by administering nicotine by means of chewing gum, skin patches, or a nasal spray. A popular product in Scandinavia consists of small sachets containing tobacco, known as 'snus' which are chewed in the oral cavity, although there have been claims that these increase the risk of oral cancers. The success of 'electronic cigarettes' which deliver nicotine but contain no tobacco is a new phenomenon. It is too early to judge whether snus or electronic cigarettes represent a safe way of quitting cigarette smoking. Even with such aids about 80 per cent of those trying to stop smoking will fall back into the habit within six months; without nicotine treatment the figure is more than 90 per cent. Some believe that the reason that smokers need to consume an average of 15–20 cigarettes a day is that they need to keep smoking to stave off the signs of tolerance and withdrawal. It is clear that nicotine is an addictive drug.

Caffeine

Caffeine, the mild stimulant present in tea and coffee, and in cola and other soft drinks, is one of the most widely and frequently consumed drugs in the world. Coffee is second only to oil as an internationally traded commodity and more than ten million people are employed in its production and marketing. Worldwide the consumption of caffeine is estimated to be approximately 70 mg per person per day—equivalent to a cup of coffee for every person on earth each day (see Figure 10). A cup of tea contains on average about half of this amount of caffeine, and a cola drink around 50 mg. There is also a variety of over-the-counter medicines or 'performance-enhancing' drinks that contain larger quantities of caffeine and are recommended to 'relieve tiredness and help maintain mental alertness'. There is some evidence that young people may misuse such caffeine-rich drinks to counteract the effects of alcohol, or that students may use them to enhance their revision or examination performance.

There have been many studies in human subjects that confirm that caffeine does indeed increase alertness and decrease fatigue. Performance on simple tasks that require sustained attention is improved, and the effect is most marked in subjects whose performance has been impaired by tiredness. Most people seem to be very good at controlling their caffeine consumption to maximize these beneficial effects, taking most caffeine when they require alertness and often avoiding caffeine later in the day to prevent sleep disturbance, although some caffeine users may suffer insomnia.

Caffeine acts as an antagonist at receptors in the brain for one of the chemical messengers called adenosine. The adenosine receptors in turn help to regulate the release of a variety of other chemical messengers. One explanation for the stimulant effects of the drug is that by blocking the normal braking actions of

The Vertue of the *COFFEE* Drink.

Firſt publiquely made and ſold in England, by *Paſqua Roſee.*

THE Grain or Berry called *Coffee*, groweth upon little Trees, only in the *Deſerts of Arabia.*

It is brought from thence, and drunk generally throughout all the Grand Seigniors Dominions.

It is a ſimple innocent thing, compoſed into a Drink, by being dryed in an Oven, and ground to Powder, and boiled up with Spring water, and about half a pint of it to be drunk, faſting an hour before, and not Eating an hour after, and to be taken as hot as poſſibly can be endured; the which will never fetch the skin off the mouth, or raiſe any Bliſters, by reaſon of that Heat.

The Turks drink at meals and other times, is uſually *Water*, and their Dyet conſiſt much of *Fruit*; the *Crudities* whereof are very much corrected by this Drink.

The quality of this Drink is cold and Dry; and though it be a Dryer, yet it neither *heats* nor *inflames* more then *hot Poſſet.*

It ſo cloſeth the Orifice of the Stomack, and fortifies the heat within it, is very good to help digeſtion; and therefore of great uſe to be bout 3 or 4 a Clock afternoon, as well as in the morning.

uen quickens the *Spirits*, and makes the Heart *Lightſome.*

is good againſt ſore Eys, and the better if you hold your Head over it, and take in the Steem that way.

It ſuppreſſeth Fumes exceedingly, and therefore good againſt the *Head-ach*, and will very much ſtop any *Defluxion of Rheums*, that diſtil from the *Head* upon the *Stomack*, and ſo prevent and help *Conſumptions*; and the *Cough of the Lungs.*

It is excellent to prevent and cure the *Dropſy, Gout*, and *Scurvy.*

It is known by experience to be better then any other Drying Drink for *People in years*, or *Children* that have any *running humors* upon them, as the *Kings Evil.* &c.

It is very good to prevent *Miſ-carryings in Child-bearing Women.*

It is a moſt excellent Remedy againſt the *Spleen*, *Hypocondriack Winds*, or the like.

It will prevent *Drowſineſs*, and make one fit for buſines, if one have occaſion to *Watch*; and therefore you are not to Drink of it *after Supper*, unleſs you intend to be *watchful*, for it will hinder ſleep for 3 or 4 hours.

It is obſerved that in Turkey, where this is generally drunk, that they are not trobled with the *Stone*, *Gout*, *Dropſie*, or *Scurvey*, and that their Skins are exceeding cleer and white.

It is neither *Laxative* nor *Reſtringent.*

Made and Sold in St. *Michaels Alley* in *Cornhill*, by *Paſqua Roſee*, at the Signe of his own Head.

10. **First-known advert for coffee (1660).**

adenosine the drug promotes more release of the chemicals acetylcholine and dopamine, both of which have stimulant effects on brain function.

Despite its apparently benign profile, however, there is evidence that chronic caffeine use can lead to a mild form of addiction. Withdrawal of caffeine from regular users leads to increased fatigue, severe headaches, and impaired performance on simple mental tasks. One school of thought even suggests that one of the reasons why people continue to take coffee, tea, or other caffeine-containing drinks during the day is not so much to improve alertness but to stave off the otherwise unpleasant signs of caffeine withdrawal—in much the same way that cigarette-smokers continue to smoke. Given the widespread and relatively uncontrolled use of caffeine, it is surprising that more research has not been devoted to answering the question of how common caffeine addiction is, or whether it represents a serious public health problem.

Cannabis

Cannabis (known as marijuana in the USA) is the most widely used of all the illegal recreational drugs. Although it has been employed for thousands of years in Asia and the Middle East both as a medicine and as a recreational drug, it is only since the 1960s and 1970s that the recreational use of cannabis has become common in the Western world. As many as a third of the population aged 15–50 in most Western countries will admit to having tried cannabis at least once, and 10–15 per cent of this age group are regular users. The definition of a 'regular user', however, covers a wide range, from those who take the drug every day to those who indulge once a month or less.

'Marijuana' or 'cannabis' are the terms used to describe the dried leaves and flowering heads of the cannabis plant. Raphael Mechoulam and his colleagues in the Hebrew University in Jerusalem during the 1970s showed that the principal psychoactive ingredient in the plant is the complex chemical Δ^9 tetrahydrocannabinol (THC). This accounts for approximately 3–4 per cent of the dry weight of the herbal material, although modern strains of the plant grown indoors under intensive cultivation conditions may contain as much as 10–15 per cent THC. Such potent forms of marijuana, known as 'skunk', represent the majority of street sales in the UK—grown locally in illegal 'cannabis farms'. Marijuana is most commonly smoked in cigarettes (joints) or in pipes of various types. Just as cigarette smoking is a very efficient way of delivering nicotine, smoking marijuana delivers THC rapidly to the smoker's brain. By adjusting smoking behaviour, the user can learn to titrate accurately the desired dose of THC. THC is also absorbed when taken by mouth, but this is a less reliable route—the absorption is slow (taking as long as 3–4 hours to reach peak blood levels) and users have no control over whether they will suffer from an overdose or a less than effective dose.

The acute intoxicant effects of cannabis are not unlike those caused by alcohol: users feel a relief of anxiety and often laugh or giggle uncontrollably. Cannabis has its own peculiar effects in distorting the sense of time (so that one minute seems much longer). At high doses it can cause hallucinations and strange fantasies and users can no longer hold a coherent conversation. There is commonly a sudden stimulation of appetite, particularly for sweet foods. These effects may be followed by tiredness and sleep.

A major advance in our understanding of how cannabis works has been the discovery that there is a specific receptor protein in the brain that recognizes THC. But why should nerve cells in our brain possess a receptor that recognizes THC—a chemical found only in the cannabis plant? The answer is that the receptors are there because the brain contains and releases its own THC-like chemical messengers, which normally activate these receptors. The naturally occurring cannabis-like chemicals are fatlike molecules; the first substance to be discovered is called 'anandamide', from the Sanskrit word for bliss, but it has been followed by several other endocannabinoids. These discoveries have had a major impact on the way in which researchers view THC and other cannabinoid drugs. Research in this field started in an attempt to discover how a plant-derived psychoactive drug worked in the brain—but this research has revealed a hitherto unrecognized naturally occurring chemical communication system in the brain. What the normal physiological function of this cannabinoid system is remains unclear, but there are strong clues that among other things it plays an important role in modulating sensitivity to pain.

The effects of cannabis on pain mechanisms probably underlie the medical uses of the drug. A medically approved cannabis extract ('Sativex') has been used in controlled clinical trials that confirm its value in treating pain and spasticity associated with multiple sclerosis (MS). Many thousands of patients in the USA and Europe prefer herbal marijuana. In Europe many patients are willing to break the law and to risk arrest and the possibility of stern punishments. In the United States twenty-three states have legalized 'cannabis pharmacies' which can dispense marijuana with a doctor's prescription, and this is also the case in Canada. The diseases for which patients most commonly report beneficial effects of cannabis are AIDS, MS, spasticity, and various conditions of chronic pain. Patients with AIDS who use marijuana report that it stimulates appetite and helps to reduce or counteract the loss of body weight, findings that are supported by clinical trial data with medicinal THC ('Marinol').

Official attitudes to cannabis have changed considerably since the 1930s, when newspapers in several major American cities ran scare stories about the new 'killer drug'. Alarm about the dangers of marijuana led the US Congress, almost by default, to pass the Marijuana Tax Act in 1937, which effectively banned the further medical use of marijuana and classed it as a dangerous narcotic.

This was later reaffirmed by the classification of marijuana in international treaties as a Schedule 1 drug—that is, a dangerous narcotic with no medical uses. Although there is a large literature on the question of how dangerous a drug cannabis is, it is often confused and lacking in the objectivity we normally expect in science. Nevertheless it is possible to summarize some of the issues in this debate.

It is clear that in the state of acute cannabis intoxication users are not capable of any work that has intellectual demands, and they should not be driving, flying an aeroplane, or operating complex machinery. Unlike alcohol, however, there are virtually no examples of people dying from an overdose of cannabis, nor is there any evidence that the drug provokes aggressive or criminal behaviour. If taken in too large a dose, however, cannabis can precipitate psychosis, characterized by paranoia.

Long-term regular users of cannabis show subtle deficits in higher brain function. In scientific terms we would refer to these as disorders in 'executive brain function'—meaning a reduced ability to remember recent events and to collate and use this information in planning future actions. Such functions are thought to involve regions of the frontal lobe of the brain, an area that is particularly rich in cannabinoid receptors. There have been concerns that these cognitive deficits might persist after cannabis use was stopped—that is, that the drug might cause permanent damage to the brain. But such fears do not appear to be well founded; nearly all of the studies of this topic have found that the cognitive deficits are completely or largely reversible.

A possible long-term health hazard in smoking cannabis concerns the risks inherent in the smoke itself. Comparisons of the smoke from cannabis and from tobacco cigarettes have shown that they contain a similar mixture of toxic chemicals. Moreover, cannabis smokers deposit 4–5 times more tar in their lungs (per joint) than cigarette-smokers. Like tobacco-smokers, cannabis smokers are liable to develop an irritating cough and signs of bronchitis. There is as yet no evidence that cannabis smoking is associated with an increased risk of lung cancer, although it may take a very long time for respiratory cancers to reveal themselves.

Cannabis is a powerful psychoactive drug and some regular users become dependent on it. Although its addictive potential seems low, the drug can come to play a dominant role in the lives of such people—and this is likely to impair their ability to function fully in their work or social life.

A debate has raged in Europe about the possibility that teenage use of cannabis can lead to psychotic illness, including schizophrenia, in later life. While a clear association exists between the early use of cannabis and the later development of schizophrenia, it will never be possible to prove a cause and effect relationship.

Some governments have concluded that the harms associated with cannabis appear to be relatively mild, and the drug should be legalized and controlled in the same way as alcohol and nicotine. Cannabis has been legalized in the Netherlands for more than forty years, and more recently in five states in the USA (Colorado, Washington, District of Columbia in Washington DC, Oregon, and Alaska). It has been 'decriminalized' in Spain, Portugal, Italy, and Czech Republic. Although it is too early to assess the consequences of legalization in some US Sates, the results of this experiment will be closely watched.

In the early years of the new millennium we have reached an interesting stage in the cannabis debate in the Western world. We must soon decide whether to reintroduce it into our medicine cabinets, and whether to accept, albeit grudgingly, that the recreational use of cannabis has become part of our culture. Our current official attitude to the drug as a dangerous narcotic comparable to cocaine and heroin is simply not compatible with what we know about the relatively modest hazards of marijuana use.

The changing attitudes to cannabis are epitomized by the publication of a series of six editorials in the *New York Times* in July 2014, making the case for legalization by addressing the social costs, racist history, and wasted resources from cannabis prohibition. The decision by America's most reputable paper to support legalization shows recognition of the powerful evidence in favour of legalization, and the shift in status quo towards radical changes in drug policies.

Amphetamines, LSD, and ecstasy

Amphetamine is one of the first man-made recreational drugs. It was first synthesized in 1887, but was tested in humans only in the 1920s. It was marketed initially as a nasal decongestant (Benzedrine), and also found medical use in the treatment of asthma and as an appetite-suppressant to treat obesity. It is a powerful stimulant though, and the side effect of sleepless nights limited its medical usefulness. This property was precisely the reason that the military started the first non-medical use of the drug during World War II, to keep pilots and other military personnel awake and alert during long missions. The dumping of large amounts of surplus amphetamine and the even more potent derivative methamphetamine (speed) by the American forces in Japan at the end of the war led to the first epidemic of widespread abuse, with up to a million users in Japan in the early 1950s. Some of the consequences soon became apparent, as many heavy users developed a form of madness ('amphetamine psychosis') that closely resembled an acute attack of schizophrenia. Fortunately the drug-induced madness usually proved reversible when drug use was stopped.

Scientifically this turned out to be a very important observation, as the way in which amphetamine acts in the brain is selectively to target those nerve cells that use the messenger molecule dopamine, and to promote an abnormally high rate of release of dopamine in the brain. As we have seen, patients with Parkinson's disease who receive an overdose of L-DOPA can also experience psychotic side effects, and these too are due to an excess of dopamine. The occurrence of amphetamine psychosis in amphetamine addicts helped to point to dopamine as a key to understanding schizophrenic illness, and to the discovery that all effective anti-schizophrenic drugs act as dopamine blockers (see Chapter 3).

The recreational use of amphetamine and methamphetamine and other amphetamine-like stimulants is very common, with as many as thirty million regular users worldwide, making this group of drugs the second most widely used after cannabis. A variant has been the use of a methamphetamine-free base ('ice'), a form of the drug that can be smoked. As with many other psychoactive drugs, smoking provides almost instant delivery to the brain and users find this especially pleasurable. Methamphetamine users also commonly inject the drug, which also causes instant gratification but may also lead to intense paranoia, and a very unpleasant comedown.

Paradoxically, amphetamine and the amphetamine-like drug methylphenidate (Ritalin) have been found to be useful in treating children with 'attention deficit hyperactivity disorder' (ADHD). These children are hyperactive and cannot attend to anything for more than a short period of time. Consequently they have difficulty in school and usually have poor academic performance. Amphetamine and methylphenidate improve the children's ability to focus their attention and to learn. There is no doubt that these drugs have beneficial effects in some children, although there is a lively debate about whether they are being overprescribed. As many as one American child in ten is said to suffer from some degree of ADHD. There is also the difficult question of whether and when the use of these stimulant drugs can be stopped as children reach adulthood. An adult form of ADHD has now been recognized.

Amphetamine or methamphetamine are relatively easy chemicals to make—anyone with a basic knowledge of chemistry and the right starting materials can make it in his or her garage or kitchen—and indeed there was a proliferation of methamphetamine labs in the USA in the 1990s. This led to the banning of the cold remedy pseudoephedrine, used as a key ingredient for methamphetamine synthesis. It is also fairly easy to make a large number of chemical variants of amphetamine, and several hundred such chemicals have been made and tested in human subjects, notably by the American chemist Alexander Shulgin and his wife—who synthesized more than one hundred amphetamine analogues—and tested them on themselves. One variant was a derivative of methamphetamine, methylene-dioxy-methamphetamine, commonly known as 'ecstasy'. Its popularity as a recreational drug coincided with the rise of the rave dance era of the 1990s. Ecstasy combines the stimulant and alerting effects of amphetamine with euphoriant and mild hallucinogenic properties, probably due to its ability to stimulate serotonin release as well as dopamine in the brain . Ecstasy was freely available until the mid-1980s, when it was made illegal on both sides of the Atlantic. Following the ban on ecstasy, a number of designer amphetamines, popularly known as 'legal highs', which lay for a while outside the drug laws, became popular. An example of these is mephedrone, a simple analogue of methamphetamine that grew rapidly in popularity in Europe in 2009–10, before it was made illegal. It has been followed by waves of novel psychoactive drugs from Chinese laboratories, which mimic the effects of amphetamine, ecstasy, LSD, opiates, or cannabis whilst remaining within the law. In recent years new synthetic drugs of this type have arrived in Europe and the USA at a rate of more than two each week—posing formidable problems for control. Despite being illegal, ecstasy remains popular in Western Europe and the USA. It is not without danger: every year the newspapers carry tragic stories of young people who die as a result of taking the drug; the number of fatalities is, however, very small by comparison with its widespread consumption. The introduction of the 'Psychoactive

Substances Bill' (2015) in Britain will make all psychoactive substances that are not already controlled illegal.

Ecstasy bears a clear chemical resemblance to amphetamine, but it also resembles the hallucinogenic compound mescaline, which is the active ingredient of the mescal cactus, used by Mexican Indians for many centuries in religious rites. Mescaline was discovered by the West as one of the first hallucinogens, and the experience was brilliantly described by Aldous Huxley (see Box 5).

Box 5 Aldous Huxley's mescaline experience

'I took my pill at eleven. An hour and a half later I was sitting in my study, looking at a small glass vase. The case contained only three flowers—a full-blown Belle of Portugal rose, shell pink with a hint at every petal's base of a hotter flamier hue; a large magenta and cream-coloured carnation; and, pale purple at the end of its broken stalk, the bold heraldic blossom of an iris. At breakfast that morning I had been struck by the lively dissonance of its colours. But that was no longer the point. I was not looking now at an unusual flower arrangement. I was seeing what Adam had seen on the morning of his creation—the miracle, moment by moment, of naked existence ... a bunch of flowers shining with their own inner light and all but quivering under the pressure of the significance with which they were charged ... I continued to look at the flowers, and in their living light I seemed to detect the qualitative equivalent of breathing—but of a breathing without returns to a starting point, with no recurrent ebbs but only a repeated flow from beauty to heightened beauty, from deeper to ever deeper meaning. Words like Grace and Transfiguration came to my mind.'

Huxley, *The Doors of Perception* (1953)

Nowadays mescaline has fallen out of favour, but the more potent hallucinogen d-LSD remains very popular (see Chapter 1). Like ecstasy, LSD is closely associated with rave dance culture. The drug interacts potently with particular serotonin receptors in the brain to cause intense auditory and visual distortions and hallucinations. It is so powerful that the human dose is about a quarter of one milligram (one-thousandth of a gram). The drug is usually dispensed as a drop of drug solution dried onto a small piece of blotting paper, which is swallowed. There is little evidence that LSD users become dependent on continuing supplies of the drug, but there can be adverse effects. Not all LSD experiences are pleasurable—the 'bad trip' can be an intensely unpleasant and frightening affair. Aldous Huxley experienced such 'bad trips' with LSD, and described his disillusionment with these drugs in his book, *Heaven and Hell* (1956).

Heroin and cocaine

In the debate about 'hard' and 'soft' recreational drugs, there is little doubt that heroin and cocaine are regarded as hard drugs. But attitudes in the West have changed over the centuries. As we have seen, opium was widely available and used in the 19th century both for medical and for recreational purposes. It was not until late in that century that restriction was first placed on its use, as the problem of addiction was recognized. Cocaine also enjoyed a brief vogue in the 1890s after it was first isolated as a pure compound from coca leaves. Cocaine was incorporated into a number of freely available tonic 'coca-wines' (Figure 2) and as an ingredient in the original Coca Cola®, until its dangers were recognized. Powder cocaine, insufflated into the nose, has seen renewed popularity among all sections of society, with a cheap poor quality drug (10–20 per cent pure) sold to a mass market, while the more affluent are offered a more expensive product of higher purity (70–80 per cent) (ACMD 2015).

Heroin

The powerful natural drug morphine from the opium poppy was a mainstay of medicine for many centuries. Heroin is a synthetic chemical derivative of morphine. It is more potent than the parent drug and it enters the brain from the blood stream more readily. This, together with the preferred route of injecting it into a vein, makes heroin the drug of choice for recreational users. Heroin users describe the 'rush' of intense euphoria and the 'high' that follows intravenous heroin as intensely pleasurable. The intensity of the intravenous heroin high makes heroin use very likely to lead to dependence and physical addiction. Withdrawal from heroin is an unpleasant and potentially life-threatening experience, with liability to diarrhoea, painful stomach cramps, headache, nausea and vomiting, and possibly convulsions. These physical signs are accompanied by an intense craving for the drug. Heroin addiction is an appalling condition: in addition to the hazards inherent in the drug itself, users are likely to die from overdose because the street drug is of variable potency and quality and at high doses the drug depresses respiration; they also run the risk of infection with hepatitis or the AIDS virus HIV because they tend to share the needles used by other addicts to inject the drug. They will develop tolerance and require ever-increasing amounts of the drug to satisfy their craving.

Like morphine, heroin acts on specific 'opiate' receptors in the brain. As in the case with cannabis, these receptors are not there to recognize the plant product. Instead they recognize a family of naturally occurring messenger molecules in the brain, the 'endorphins' (see Chapter 3). There are several different endorphins and at least three distinct types of opiate receptors, but one in particular—the 'mu-opioid receptor' (MOR) seems to be responsible both for the pain-relieving and the pleasurable effects of morphine and heroin. Mice that are genetically engineered so that they do not express MOR in their brain no longer seek out the drug, and it has no pain-relieving actions in such animals.

The use of heroin is unfortunately on the increase, particularly in deprived inner-city areas both in Europe and in the USA. The drug is supplied by well-organized international criminal cartels, using opium from poppies grown as a profitable cash crop in Asia and South America. A modern version of heroin use involves smoking pure heroin as an alternative to injection, a method known as 'chasing the dragon'. Again smoking has proved to be a rapid and effective means of getting the drug quickly to the receptors in the brain—and at least this removes the risk associated with dirty needles.

Treatments for heroin addiction usually involve giving the addict the substitute opiate drug, methadone. This is taken by mouth, is absorbed slowly, and has a long-lasting effect. Without giving the 'high' of heroin it helps to stave off the craving for the drug. Although methadone clinics have had some success, it is difficult to persuade addicts to stop taking heroin. Our society also continues to emphasize the punishment of drug addicts as criminals, rather than as unfortunate individuals in need of medical treatment. To prevent recurrence, the opiate receptor antagonist naltrexone has proved of some use; it prevents the pleasurable effects of the drug. Another opiate antagonist naloxone is also a valuable 'rescue' medicine, capable of reversing otherwise fatal heroin overdoses, and is being made more generally available to paramedics, and to family members and friends (ACMD, 2013). Needle exchange centres can reduce the harm associated with injected drugs. Heroin overdose is the commonest form of drug-related death—the 'window' between the desired intoxicant effects and respiratory depression is narrow, and even experienced addicts can misjudge the dose.

Cocaine

Like morphine, cocaine is a plant product, produced in the leaves of the coca plant—grown particularly in the South American Andes. The huge increase in demand for cocaine as a recreational drug has led to the development of a highly profitable illegal export business for several South American and Latin American countries. In the case of Colombia, this business has virtually destroyed the fabric of society and the maintenance of law and order.

Cocaine is usually taken by insufflating (sniffing) the white powdered cocaine sulphate into the nose, which leads to rapid absorption of the drug into the bloodstream. A modern variant uses a form of cocaine base ('crack cocaine'), which is smoked or injected—giving an even more rapid and intensely pleasurable 'high'. Those who have experienced the cocaine high describe it as the most powerful of all drug-induced pleasures. Animals seem to agree (they will rapidly learn to self-administer the drug) and, if given unlimited access, will continue to self-administer to the detriment of all other behaviours—including feeding, drinking, and sex. Crack cocaine is the ultimate drug of addiction: it is estimated that 10–15 per cent of people who experiment with crack cocaine are destined to become regular users. Cocaine addiction seems to be a miserable form of existence. The cocaine high is often followed by a deep depression of mood and the ever-constant need to find the next dose of drug to relieve this black mood. The addict may lack all motivation except to seek further supplies of the drug, and will often steal or murder to obtain these. The use of cocaine doubled or trebled in many countries during the 1990s and has remained at this new high level. Closer analysis, however, has shown that the rise in cocaine use can almost entirely be accounted for by a rise in the use of powder cocaine. In the UK a two-tier market for powder cocaine has developed, with at one end cheap low-purity material (10–20 per cent cocaine plus 'fillers') and at the other more expensive high-grade material (80–90 per cent cocaine). Users of powder cocaine tend to take the drug infrequently, and probably run a low risk of addiction (ACMD, 2014).

In the brain cocaine acts to promote the serotonin, the norepinephrine, and the dopamine systems. It does so by acting as an inhibitor of the transporters that are responsible for the uptake of these chemical messengers. This combined pharmacology gives the combined stimulant and arousing effect of amphetamine with the mood-elevating action of Prozac.

Drugs and the law

The regulation of the availability of recreational drugs through legislation has proved to be a very confusing area. While most people would agree that some restrictions need to be placed on the availability of potentially dangerous drugs, particularly to young people, it is less easy to understand why some drugs should be restricted (for example, alcohol) and others banned altogether. Some have described drug taking as a 'victimless crime': who is being damaged other than the users themselves? However, the danger to others of drunk driving is well understood, and the increased incidence of drivers intoxicated with various psychoactive drugs has lead to the introduction of kerbside drug testing in the UK.

Most Western countries have agreed to an international criminal code, which covers many illicit recreational drugs, by means of a series of United Nations conventions framed in the 1960s and 1970s. Most countries operate their own classification system for illicit drugs within this UN framework. In Britain the Misuse of Drugs Act (1971) places drugs in three categories, A, B, and C, with decreasing scales of punishment for criminal offences. The schedules are as follows:

A. Cocaine, ecstasy, LSD, morphine, heroin, opium
B. Amphetamines, barbiturates, cannabis, methamphetamine, codeine

C. Anabolic steroids, benzodiazepines, pemoline, phentermine, mazindol, diethylpropion

The problem is that, despite the expenditure of large efforts on both sides of the Atlantic in the so-called 'War on Drugs', the war has not been won. Indeed, the abuse of drugs is continuing to increase and the criminal underworld that supplies this apparently insatiable demand is flourishing. There are no easy solutions in sight. There are more than half a million cannabis-related arrests in the USA every year, and some 70,000 in Britain—representing in each case more than half of all drug-related offences. Surely police time and resources would be better devoted to really dangerous drugs such as cocaine and heroin? When young people can see that the law is unfair, they come to disrespect it. The Dutch experiment of making small quantities of cannabis freely available in a system of 'coffee shops' has not led to the breakdown of Dutch society—nor do rates of cannabis consumption in Holland differ from those elsewhere in the Western world. The Dutch claim, however, that they have successfully separated the source of cannabis from that of other more dangerous drugs and their problem with heroin and other 'hard drugs' is lessening. Sooner or later politicians will have to learn to take the scientific and medical evidence more seriously. Too much of the drug debate has been ill-informed and demonized.

Societal changes in attitude to recreational drugs do occasionally happen. When pure cocaine was first discovered it was a popular ingredient in health products; it is no longer. Morphine, or opium, were essential ingredients in 19th-century medicines—but are now regarded as highly dangerous. Cigarette smoking, once seen a valuable health aid, is now taboo. Attitudes to cannabis have softened, with moves to legalize or decriminalize use of the drug on both sides of the Atlantic.

Chapter 5
Making new medicines

The discovery, development, and marketing of new prescription medicines has become a major worldwide industry. Pharmaceutical companies, focused mainly in the USA, Western Europe, and Japan (but now growing rapidly in China and India also), have become an important component of the economies of many nations. Some of the individual companies are among the largest and wealthiest in any industry, employing tens of thousands of staff and enjoying annual revenues amounting in total to around $1 trillion worldwide. The successful discovery and marketing of a new medicine can also be a very profitable business, with annual sales of 'blockbuster' drugs often in excess of $1 billion and carrying a high profit margin.

Such returns are always transitory though; there will always be a competitor coming along with a similar medicine willing to undercut in price. The pharmaceutical industry relies heavily on patents to protect its products, so that a competitor cannot immediately sell the same medicine, but a competitor can market a similar product that lies outside the scope of the original patent. Patents also have finite lives and the twenty years of protection usually provided by a patent are often substantially eroded during the long process of research and development (R&D) needed before a product can come to market. After the patent expires, any company can copy the

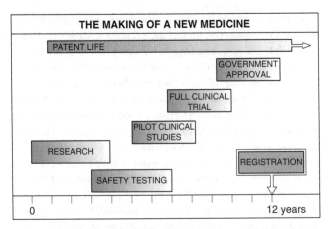

11. **The making of a new medicine involves a number of time-consuming stages. Overall the process from laboratory bench to doctor's desk can take more than ten years.**

drug and market it as a so-called 'generic' product, and this has created a secondary industry of companies that specialize in the production and marketing of generic medicines. As they do not have to incur the expensive costs of R&D, the generic drug companies can market the product much more cheaply than the original discoverer. Because new products have only a finite commercial life, the major companies must always be looking for the next generation of medicines, preferably the new blockbusters. How this is done has become an extraordinarily complex and high-tech process (see Figure 11).

Drug discovery

All drugs act on specific receptors (see Chapter 2) and most innovative companies seek to discover new receptor targets that offer a novel approach to the treatment of a particular disease. The range of new targets available is being extended greatly as our knowledge of the human genome becomes increasingly complete.

Humans have around 30,000–40,000 genes, each of which encodes the information for making a protein. Clearly not all of these will be suitable drug targets, but many new targets will emerge. Most of the medicines available in the 20th century targeted one or other of the surface membrane receptor proteins or ion channels then known. We now know that there are 2,000 or more such potential drug targets. In addition some drugs target enzymes, usually as inhibitors. For example, the family of protein kinase enzymes, which add phosphate groups to cell proteins, numbers hundreds of sub-species, many of which play a critical role in cell division, and the growth inhibitors of specific kinase inhibitors have proved valuable in the treatment of cancer (Table 2). The problem for companies is how to decide which of the many possible novel targets offer the greatest chance of providing effective new treatments, and which ones to invest in. New targets will, nevertheless, be found that offer novel approaches to treating diseases, based on new knowledge of the disease process.

Once a target has been chosen, a number of panels of human cell surface receptor, ion channels, transporters, and enzymes such as kinases or cytochrome P450 variants, are available for the testing of large numbers of new drug candidates. The synthesis of new drug chemicals as candidates for screening used to be a laborious and slow process. Each new chemical was made individually by expert chemists, who on average could produce one or two new compounds each week. Since the 1990s, however, this process has been radically changed by the introduction of robot chemistry, which allows the assembly of the various chemical constituents that make up new drug molecules in many different permutations. Using such 'combinatorial chemistry' techniques, a single chemist can now produce thousands of new compounds each week. Specialized companies have emerged that synthesize chemical libraries containing hundreds of thousands or even millions of new chemicals and sell them to pharmaceutical companies for their own particular screening projects. The screening of large numbers of new chemicals has become possible because of the parallel development of new 'high throughput' screening technology. By using robot laboratories capable of handling very large numbers of tests and using computers to store the mass of data that result, it is now possible for a company to screen as many as a million new chemicals in less than one month against a given target, or against multiple targets. This process of mass screening should generate a number of 'lead' chemicals with some activity at the target receptor. By examining the chemical features that the lead structures have in common, chemists can then further refine these leads to create improved drug candidates with even stronger actions on the target receptor.

The large-scale screening involves simple tests on the human receptor target in a test tube or cell culture model. The next stage will involve testing the best drug candidates in more complex biological systems, often using the isolated organs or tissues of experimental animals, or cell lines expressing human target receptors for in vitro pharmacology. The shortlisted candidates may then be tested by giving them to living animals. In some cases this is the only way of testing the effectiveness of new drug candidates—for example in assessing the effects of drugs on animal behaviour in tests that predict new antidepressant or anti-schizophrenic medicines.

Monoclonal antibodies

More than a hundred years ago Paul Ehrlich proposed the idea of a 'magic bullet' postulating that a compound could be made that selectively targets a disease-causing organism. The monoclonal antibody is the closest we have come to the 'magic bullet', and this relatively new class of medicines is having a major impact in treating hitherto untreatable conditions.

When an organism is exposed to an antigen, the immune system responds by generating thousands of different antibodies. In order to be useful as medicines a single antibody must be isolated.

In the original procedure, discovered by Kohler and Milstein, mice are injected with an antigen and the antibody-forming cells are isolated from the spleen; these cells do not divide, but they are then fused with cells of a myeloma cancer cell line, to form 'hybridomas' which will divide and multiply in tissue culture. The hybridoma expressing an antibody with the highest affinity for binding the antigen can be selected out, and will grow and divide indefinitely, and will secrete the monoclonal antibody. Because the hybridoma has been immortalized by fusion with the cancer cell line (myeloma) it can be grown in large amounts from a single clone to generate 'monoclonal antibody' medicines (see Figure 12).

Nowadays not all monoclonal antibody production depends on using mice to generate antibodies. The most commonly used technique called 'phage display' involves the production of libraries of bacteriophages (viruses which infect bacteria), in which each phage expresses one human antibody. Such libraries, displaying many thousands of different antibodies, are readily generated and can even be obtained commercially. By passing the phage library through a column of material to which the antigen has been attached, the phages binding with high affinity to the antigen will become attached, and can then be isolated and amplified to generate monoclonal antibodies.

The medical importance of monoclonal antibodies has stimulated a great deal of research aimed at further improvements. Antibodies generated in mice will be rejected as 'foreign' proteins by the body, so methods have been developed to 'humanize' them by replacing parts of the mouse antibody with human antibody fragments. Another method of producing human antibodies is to use mice that are genetically engineered to express human rather than murine antibodies. Other improvements have aimed to yield antibodies with longer lifetimes in human subjects. Monoclonal antibodies have also been coupled to reagents that will extend their toxicity—for example coupling to a radioactive or other

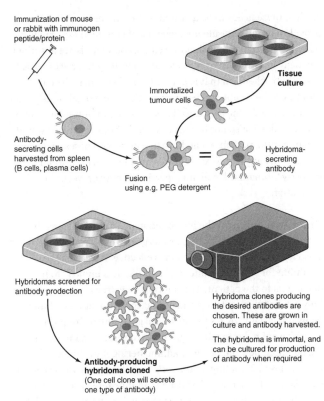

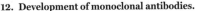

12. **Development of monoclonal antibodies.**

cytotoxic fragment that allows the monoclonal antibody to destroy cancer cells after it has bound selectively to them.

Drug development

The initial screening may involve hundreds of antibodies, or thousands of synthetic chemicals, but this will have been reduced to a shortlist for assessment in the whole-animal tests. From these, a handful of possible development candidates will emerge.

Each of these needs to be assessed to see whether it is likely to provide a useful and safe medicine. Further animal experiments will be needed to establish how well the compounds are absorbed when given by mouth or injected, and how long their actions last. A synthetic chemical that is not well absorbed when given by mouth will be troublesome unless another route of administration can be devised. One that is well absorbed but rapidly degraded or eliminated will also not be attractive, as in human use this would mean that the patient would have to take several doses each day. Monoclonal antibodies are administered by injection, and if properly 'humanized' will often persist for days or weeks in circulation.

To obtain approval for the introduction of a new medicine, the company needs to satisfy the various government regulatory agencies both that the compound is effective in treating the condition for which it is intended and that it is unlikely to be dangerous to the patient. The safety of new drugs can never be fully predicted by tests in animals, but these can at least eliminate many potentially toxic substances. All governments require extensive animal safety testing. This involves, for example, testing the potential new medicine by administering it to animals at various doses, including at least one high dose greatly in excess of any planned human use. The drug is administered every day for periods of up to two years. During this period the animals will be weighed regularly and blood samples taken to see whether any biochemical or blood abnormalities are triggered. At the end of the test period the animals are killed and their various internal organs visually examined and weighed and then examined in detail under the microscope to detect any possible adverse changes, in particular the formation of tumours or other evidence of cancer. These safety tests will be repeated in two different mammalian species to maximize the chance of detecting any toxicity. Special animal tests in pregnant animals will be needed if the drug is to be used in women of child-bearing age—to detect any possible adverse effects that the compound might have on the developing foetus (the thalidomide tragedy was the spur to improve such tests).

The safety testing of monoclonal antibodies poses special problems. As the antibodies are human or have been 'humanized' they will produce an immune reaction if administered to mice. To overcome this, safety testing is sometimes carried out using non-human primates. But the use of such animals in research is vigorously opposed. Another approach is to test the antibody in a small group of human volunteers, using initially very low doses. This can, however, have disastrous consequences; an infamous trial of an antibody directed against the immune system protein CD28 led to multiple organ failure in the volunteers, involving an uncontrolled immune response. The use of mice genetically engineered to express human antibodies offers a safer approach, and assessment of renal, cardiac, and other required safety tests can readily be done.

Provided the development compound passes these safety tests, it can then be administered to human subjects for the first time. The initial Phase 1 clinical trials involve a small number of healthy volunteers. They receive the drug under carefully monitored conditions to make sure that it does not cause any unpredicted, unpleasant, or dangerous side effects. Monitoring drug or antibody levels in blood samples from such volunteers will also provide valuable information on how well the drug is absorbed in humans, how long it persists in the body, and what the main breakdown products are. This information will help the selection of the most suitable dose regime for the next stage (Phase 2) of clinical tests, which involve patients. These trials are usually done with small numbers of patients, and the aim is to test whether the drug actually works—that is, does it improve the patients' symptoms? In the case of drugs that target a novel human receptor for the first time, this 'proof of concept' is particularly vital; it may not always work out the way the scientists predicted.

All clinical trials need to take account of the 'placebo' effect. Sick patients want to believe that the new medicine will help them to get better, and it is well established that many patients show a definite measurable improvement even when given a dummy (placebo) pill that does not contain any active drug. The placebo effect is particularly marked for disorders of the central nervous system; trials of new antidepressants or pain-relieving compounds will always show a placebo effect. The nature of the placebo effect remains a mystery. The strength of the placebo effect is related to the complexity of the treatment procedure. Swallowing several tablets has a more powerful effect than simply taking one, an intravenous injection is even more powerful, and treatment involving a mock surgical procedure is even better. As with many drug treatments, the effectiveness of the placebo tends to wear off with repeated administrations. The placebo effect seems to reflect the remarkable ability of the human mind to control the body, and it may well underlie the effectiveness of various 'alternative-medicine' approaches to treating illness. From the point of view of drug development, however, the placebo effect complicates the clinical assessment of new drugs. In order to see whether any beneficial effects observed in patients are due to the drug itself or simply to a placebo effect, it is necessary to compare the active drug with a placebo. This is usually accomplished in a so-called randomized double-blind placebo-controlled trial. In such trials patients are randomly allocated to groups that receive either a placebo or an active drug. Neither the patient nor the doctor or nurse administering the medicine knows whether the patient is receiving an active drug or a placebo—to avoid any possibility of suggestion. At the end of the trial the code is broken and the results analysed. Only if the drug is statistically significantly more beneficial than the placebo can the trial be called a success. The results of these trials will also help to establish whether the drug caused any adverse side effects over and above any that were observed in the placebo group. For example, it is common for patients to complain of headache or feelings of nausea, but these may not necessarily be drug related. If adverse drug-related effects are observed, these must be noted and explained to all patients receiving the compound in the future.

In the happy event that the results of the Phase 2 trials are positive, the compound can enter much larger Phase 3 clinical trials. These commonly involve hundreds or thousands of patients, recruited in a number of different medical centres—usually university medical schools and hospitals. Because of their complexity, and the need to treat patients over extended periods of time, these trials can often take years to complete. At every stage detailed records need to be kept of each patient and, wherever possible, objective methods used to measure improvement in clinical state. One may measure reductions in blood pressure or blood cholesterol, for example. In some conditions, however, particularly those involving disorders of the central nervous system, such objective measurements may not be possible—and one has to rely on the patients' own assessments of their mood, or how much pain they are feeling. In many countries regulatory agencies may require positive results in two Phase 3 clinical trials before approving the new medicine. The USA now requires companies to disclose the results of all clinical trials, to avoid the 'cherry picking' of only the positive trials.

The randomized clinical trial has become the gold standard for evaluating new drugs; the concept was only developed after the end of World War II. Nowadays the randomized trial is finding new uses in evaluating the effectiveness of social, criminal, and political processes.

Registration and marketing

If all goes well with these Phase 3 trials, the company will be ready to assemble a massive package of data. This will include a detailed description of all the results obtained on the compound in the clinic, in animal safety, and in the laboratory, together with information on how the compound can be manufactured and what quality-control measures exist. Such a package of data will occupy many volumes, nowadays stored in computer files and submitted online to a government regulatory agency for detailed scrutiny, and after expert assessment. The agency will inevitably come back to the company with a list of questions that need to be answered, often involving the need for the company to undertake further tests for efficacy or safety. After this process has been completed the agency may hold a meeting at which a panel of experts can interrogate company representatives on the fine points of their submission. The panel then votes to advise the government agency whether to approve or decline the submission. The process of review by the regulatory agency can take many months to complete, although for some diseases (for example, AIDS) there are fast-track approval procedures.

Once a new medicine has been given official registration, the company is free to market it, but it can only be recommended and advertised for the particular disorders for which official approval was given. Any additional new medical uses will need further clinical trial data and government approval before the company can promote these. After marketing has started there is a system of 'post-marketing surveillance', which requires doctors to alert the authorities to adverse drug effects. This is designed to detect any rare adverse effects that the compound may cause. Even though the clinical trials involve thousands of patients, they cannot detect rare adverse effects that may occur, for example, in only 1 in 100,000 patients. These can sometimes be serious or even life threatening, and they can lead to the rapid withdrawal of new compounds from the market—a bitter pill to swallow for the company involved. New medicines represent entirely novel chemical molecules or antibodies to which humans have never been exposed; their safety is never going to be completely predictable.

Prescription medicines are not the only medicines on the market. It is far easier to gain approval for the introduction of herbal medicines where proof of efficacy is not required. On the other hand, the company marketing a herbal medicine is also not allowed to make specific medical claims for it; the alleged benefits have to be couched in more general terms. Homeopathic medicines represent a special case, as these often involve diluting active ingredients to such an extent that there may be few or no active drug molecules remaining in the marketed preparation, the ultimate placebo medicine. Regulatory agencies have never been sure how to deal with homeopathic medicines. At the end of the day they seem to have concluded that at least they are unlikely to do patients any serious harm and their approval remains relaxed. Nevertheless, patients taking homeopathic medicines may refuse to take more effective medicines—in the case of cancer this could be life-threatening.

Chapter 6
What can we expect in the future?

Changing attitudes to drugs

While scientific discoveries continue to deliver new medicines at an ever-accelerating pace, public attitudes to drugs are changing. Patients no longer view their doctor as the fount of all wisdom. By scanning the Internet patients can obtain detailed information on the most effective treatments for their illness, and the effectiveness and side effects of prescribed medicines. Some will come to the doctor's surgery brandishing such papers! On the one hand it is good that technical knowledge about drug treatment should be freely available, on the other hand the patients may hold irrational views on drug treatment in general, and on specific treatments in particular. For example, there are campaigns in the USA and in the UK against childhood vaccination—although this has undoubtedly saved many lives in the past hundred years. Those opposed to vaccination can always find support for their beliefs from Internet sites, which promote such views. The idea that 'vaccination causes autism' remains firmly embedded on both sides of the Atlantic, despite its complete dismissal by scientific studies. In some parts of the UK and USA vaccination rates in the population have dropped below the minimum required to achieve 'herd immunity'.

Social attitudes to recreational drugs are also changing. Users question government advice on the harmfulness of drugs, and construct their own views on such matters.

For example, moves to legalize cannabis are gaining ground—despite the insistence of the UK and US governments that it is a dangerous drug.

The pharmaceutical industry

The complex and exacting process of drug discovery and development takes many years to complete and involves company scientists and outside experts from many different disciplines. The whole process from initial screening to final product often takes ten years or more and the costs involved continue to escalate as regulatory agencies set more and more demanding criteria for drug approval. On average, for every one hundred promising drug candidates discovered in the research laboratory only ten will get as far as being assessed in human subjects, and only one of these will become a registered new medicine. Even then, less than half of the new medicines will make a profit for the company. Since each new medicine costs several hundred million dollars to develop, pharmaceutical companies use the high cost of R&D to justify the high prices and profit margins they obtain for new products. Pharmaceutical companies reinvest more than 10 per cent of their income on R&D, a far higher proportion than most other sectors of industry. On the other hand, the companies operate very high profit margins, and they spend equally heavily on marketing their products, both to doctors and more recently to the individual patient, with TV adverts permitted in the USA. Stock markets expect the income of the major companies to continue to grow in every year. Those companies that fail to grow may merge or be absorbed by others who have been more successful. Each year sees the industry increasingly dominated by a smaller number of giant companies formed as the result of such mergers. The high prices that new prescription medicines command, and the profits that companies report, have given the pharmaceutical industry a poor public image in recent years. There is anger too about the fact that poor countries have often been denied the benefits of Western medicines, because the industry insists on maintaining the patent restrictions on its products throughout the world. Although governments already exert considerable regulation over the industry—for example, in setting new product prices in many countries—it seems likely that there will be pressure for even more such intervention in the future.

Meanwhile the costs of new medicines escalate. Worldwide prescription drug sales are expected to reach $1 trillion by 2020. In 2010 in the USA the cost of medicine per patient per year averaged $1,000–$2,000. By 2014 the average cost per patient year for the top ten drugs had increased to $9,180–$56,212. Some of this increase is based on the high price of monoclonal antibodies, but synthetic drugs also raised high revenues; in 2014 lenalidomide 'Revlimid' (a thalidomide analogue) treated 17,380 patients at an annual cost per patient of $164,859; everolimus 'Affinitor' (a tyrosine kinase inhibitor) treated 7,253 patients at an annual cost per patient of $106,675; and the nucleotide analogue sofosbuvir (Sovaldi®) for treatment of Hepatitis C, carries a price tag of $78,000. Two new monoclonal antibodies for the treatment of lung cancer, 'Keytruda®' and 'Opdivo®' are expected to generate sales in excess of $1 billion within a few years of launch.

The high prices demanded by US companies make new medicines too expensive for most European health services, and out of reach of developing countries. In the US, insurance companies or government schemes seem able to pay. Indeed the US Congress passed a law in 2003 banning Medicare (a Government agency that purchases prescription drugs for the elderly) from negotiating drug prices. Companies argue that new drugs for the treatment of rare diseases still have high R&D costs, and these need to be recouped. Such arguments have led most companies to abandon research on antibiotics and other anti-infective agents.

Government funding will be needed to subsidize such R&D in the future. In the UK an increasing clamour by cancer patients and their relatives for access to the new high-cost treatments has induced the UK government set aside money in a 'Cancer Fund' to meet high-priority needs, but this is at best only a palliative measure. The high prices of monoclonal antibodies will persist as long as there is no competition. Although monoclonal antibodies are not subject to 'generic' competition when patents expire, the European Drug Council has approved 'biosimilars' to compete with patent-expired monoclonals (Chapter 3)—and this may be the way forward, although this approach is not yet approved in the USA.

Patients outside the USA may have to wait until the patents on new drugs expire and cheaper 'generics' or 'biosimilars' become available. Meanwhile the looming crisis of increased resistance to most antibiotics and other anti-infective drugs is a worldwide problem that needs to be addressed urgently. Even if pharmaceutical companies could be persuaded to re-enter this field, it could take many years before new drugs become available.

Personalized medicines

As understanding of the genetic and molecular basis of diseases has increased rapidly, and the costs of DNA sequencing have plummeted, research is focusing on how to apply this new knowledge in the clinic. There is a movement towards personalized medicine, which aims to tailor treatment to an individual patient.

This approach has developed most rapidly in cancer treatments. It has generated drugs which are effective only in patients possessing specific mutations in cancer cells; thus, for example, 'Herceptin' is only effective in patients over-expressing the HER-2 protein; 'Irrisa' is only effective in treating lung cancer in patients with a mutation leading to increased expression of growth factor receptor EGFR; taflinar selectively treats melanoma which express the BRAF-V600E gene.

Thus, although still in its infancy, some medicines targeting particular mutations in cancer cells already exist. The aim will be to use DNA sequencing of cancer cells to determine the patterns of mutation and molecular pathways that lead to cancer. In future the objective is to develop individual treatments directed to such genetic information, rather than the current practice of targeting organ-specific cancers (see Table 2). Similar approaches could be used for other diseases. The implications for the pharmaceutical industry are fairly obvious. Developing multiple drugs to treat particular genetic forms of illness will be costly, and likely lead to ever-higher prices in the pharmacy.

Another aspect of the genetic assessment of individuals is to identify carriers of genes that carry a high risk of cancer or other illness. About 5-10 per cent of breast cancer may be hereditary to carriers of mutated forms of BRAC1 or BRAC2 genes. Women carrying such mutated genes have an 80 per cent risk of developing breast and/or ovarian cancer, and some will opt to have breasts and ovary removed surgically as a prophylactic measure. Here genetic information is reducing the future risk of illness, and also providing targets for new medicines.

A number of large-scale projects are underway involving many thousands of subjects to characterize the genetic make-up of cancer and other cells and to generate new understanding of the complex relation between genes, mutations, and illness.

A futuristic field of research aims to use synthetic RNAs as medicines. 'Messenger RNA' is the nucleic acid translated from DNA gene sequences which acts as the messenger between nuclear DNA and the synthesis of specific proteins. Synthetic messenger RNAs can be designed to supplement body proteins, to modify the function of the immune system, or to act as vaccines. Several examples of this new class of medicines are already being developed and are in clinical trials.

An even more futuristic idea is to target drugs at the epigenetic mechanisms that we now understand up-regulate or down-regulate gene expression.

Ending the war on drugs

The 20th century saw the 'war on drugs', with thousands of young people arrested and many imprisoned for crimes against the drug laws, which made both possession and sale of restricted recreational drugs criminal offences.

In the 21st century there is a growing realization that this approach has failed. Despite harsh criminal penalties, the sale and consumption of recreational drugs has increased, and new chemical modifications repeatedly challenge existing laws (e.g. 'legal highs').

Society's attitude to drugs has changed radically over the past two centuries: opium and cocaine from good to evil; nicotine from good to evil. Cannabis, although subject to criminal laws which lead to hundreds of thousands of arrests and imprisonments each year, is gradually being seen by many governments to be no more dangerous than alcohol or tobacco. Moves to legalize cannabis are already being made, controlling it in the same way as alcohol or tobacco. This may prove an inexorable change in attitude and law, similar to the sea change in attitudes to tobacco in the 20th century.

References

Chapter 1: History

Berridge, V., and Edwards, G., *Opium and the People* (London: St Martin Press, Allen Lane, 1981).

Culpeper, N., *Pharmacopoeia Londinensis* (1659).

Encyclopaedia Britannica (2015), 'Medicine—History of: Medicine and Surgery before 1800': <www.britannica.com>.

Hoffmann, A., 'History of the Discovery of LSD', in A. Pletscher and D. Ladweig (eds.), *50 Years of LSD* (London: Parthenon Publishing Group, 1994).

Chapter 2: How drugs work

Rang, H., Ritter, J. M., Flower, R. J., and Henderson, G., *Rang & Dale's Pharmacology*, 8th edn. (London: Elsevier Ltd., 2016).

Brunton, L. L., Parker, K. L., Blumenthal, D., and Buxt, I. (eds.), *Goodman and Gilman's Manual of Pharmacology and Therapeutics* (New York: McGraw Hill, 2007).

Chapter 3: Drugs as medicines

WHO Media Centre. Fact Sheet 194. *Antimicrobial Resistance*, updated April 2015.

O'Neill, J., *Antimicrobial Resistance: Tackling a Crisis for the Health and Wealth of Nations* (London: UK Government, 2014).

National Cancer Institute. *Targeted Cancer Therapies* <http://www.cancer.gov/cancertopics/treatment/types/targeted-therapies> (visited 23.04.2015).

Gibson, M., *The Long Strange History of Birth Control* (2015). <www.time.com/3692001/birth-control-history-djerrasi/> (visited 26.12.15).

Chapter 4: Recreational drugs

Advisory Council on the Misuse if Drugs. *Consideration of Naloxone* (2012). <https://www.gov.uk/government/publications/consideration-of-naloxone>.

Advisory Council on the Misuse of Drugs, *Cocaine Powder: Review of its Prevalence, Patterns of Use and Harm* (2015). <https://www.gov.uk/government/publications/cocaine-powder-review-of-its-prevalence-patterns-of-use-and-harm>.

Benowitz, N. L., *The Biology of Nicotine Dependence* (CIBA Foundation Symposium 152; Chichester: John Wiley & Sons, 1990).

Dargan, P., and Wood, D. M., *Novel Psychoactive Substances* (London: Academic Press, 2013).

Huxley, A., *The Doors of Perception* (London: Chatto and Windus, 1953).

Huxley, A., *Heaven and Hell* (London: Chatto and Windus, 1956).

Liu, B. Q., et al., 'Emerging Tobacco Hazards in China. I: Retrospective Proportional Mortality Study of One Million Deaths', *British Medical Journal*, 317 (1998): 1411–22.

Peto, R., et al., 'Smoking, Smoking Cessation, and Lung Cancer in the UK since 1950: Combination of National Statistics with Two Case Control Studies', *British Medical Journal*, 321 (2000): 323–9.

Chapter 5: Making new medicines

Hansel, T. T., Kropshofer, H., Sionger, T., Mitchell, J. A., and George, A. J. T., 'The Safety and Side Effects of Monoclonal Antibodies'. Nature Reviews, *Drug Discovery*, 9 (2010): 325–50.

Blass, B., *Basic Principles of Drug Discovery* (London: Elsevier, 2015).

Chapter 6: What can we expect in the future?

Breast Cancer Risk Factors: *Genetics* <http://www.breastcancer.org/risk%20factors/genetics> (visited 18.05.2015).

Shaugnessy, A., 'Monoclonal Antibodies: Magic Bullets with a Hefty Price Tag', *British Medical Journal* (2012), <http://www.bmj.com/content/345/bmj.e8346>.

Humphries C. *Cancer Treatment Gets Personal* (2013) <http://harvardmagazine.com/2013/11/cancer_treatment_gets_personal>.

Sahin, U., Kariko, K., and Tureci, O., 'mRNA-based Therapeutics—Developing a New Class of Drugs', Nature Reviews, *Drug Discovery* 13 (2014): 759–79.

Further reading

Chapter 1: History

Gerald, M. C., *The Drug Book: From Arsenic to Xanax, 250 Milestones in the History of Drugs*, Sterling Milestones (New York: Sterling, 2013).

Karlen, A., *Plagues Progress: A Social History of Man and Disease* (London: Victor Gollancz, 1995). A good account of how infectious diseases have influenced history.

Chapter 2: How drugs work

Rang, H., Ritter, J. M., Flower, R. J., and Henderson, G., *Rang & Dale's Pharmacology*, 8th edn. (London: Elsevier Ltd., 2016).

Brunton, L. L., Parker, K. L., Blumenthal, D., and Buxt, I. (eds.), *Goodman and Gilman's Manual of Pharmacology and Therapeutics* (New York: McGraw Hill, 2007).

Chapter 3: Drugs as medicines

Cancer Research UK—Official Site <https://www.cancerresearchuk.org>.

Healy, D., *The Antidepressant Era* (Cambridge, MA: Harvard University Press, 1997). A fascinating account of the history of antidepressant drugs in the 20th century, written for the non-specialist reader.

Iversen, L., *Speed, Ecstasy, Ritalin: The Science of Amphetamines* (Oxford: Oxford University Press, 2008).

Iversen, L., Iversen, S., Bloom, F., and Roth, R., *The Biochemical Basis of Psychopharmacology* (Oxford: Oxford University Press, 2008). An introduction to the mechanism of action of CNS drugs, and their use in medicine.

Stone, T., and Darlington, G., *Pills, Potions and Poisons: How Drugs Work* (Oxford: Oxford University Press, 2000). An introductory book written for the non-specialist reader.

Chapter 4: Recreational drugs

Berridge, V., *Demons: Our Changing Attitudes to Alcohol, Tobacco, and Drugs* (Oxford: Oxford University Press, 2013).

Iversen, L., *The Science of Marijuana*, 2nd edn. (New York: Oxford University Press, 2008). A review of how cannabis works and the pros and cons of its medicinal or recreational use, written for the non-specialist.

Jay, M. (2000), *Emperors of Dreams: Drugs in the Nineteenth Century* (Sawtry, Cambs.: Dedalus, 2000). A well-written account of the social history of recreational drug use in the 19th century, from laughing gas and ether to heroin and cocaine.

Robson, P., *Forbidden Drugs*, 2nd edn. (Oxford: Oxford University Press, 1999). Readable account of recreational drugs and drug abuse.

Shulgin, A., and Shulgin, A., *PiHKAL, a Chemical Love Story* (Berkeley, CA: Transform Press, 1997).

Stone, T., and Darlington, G., *Pills, Potions, and Poisons* (Oxford: Oxford University Press, 2000).

Chapter 5: Making new medicines

Warne, P., *How Drugs Are Developed: An Introduction to Pharmaceutical R&D*, SCRIP Reports (London: PJB Publications Ltd., 2003).

Chapter 6: What can we expect in the future?

Duke, S. B., *The Future of Marijuana in the United States* (2013) <http://digitalcommons.law.yale.edu/fss_papers/4842>.

Fischer, J. (ed.)., *Successful Drug Discovery, vol. 1* (Oxford: J. Wiley & Sons, 2015).

Nutt, D., Robbins, T. W., Stimson, G. V., Ince, M., and Jackson, A. (eds.), *Drugs and the Future. Brain Science, Addiction and Society* (Oxford: Elsevier, 2007).

Powledge, T. 'Behavioral Epigenetics: How Nurture Shapes Nature', *Bioscience*, 61 (2011): 588–92.

Index

Drugs